Cancer
A Beginner's Guide

ONEWORLD BEGINNER'S GUIDES combine an original, inventive, and engaging approach with expert analysis on subjects ranging from art and history to religion and politics, and everything in-between. Innovative and affordable, books in the series are perfect for anyone curious about the way the world works and the big ideas of our time.

aesthetics
africa
american politics
anarchism
ancient philosophy
animal behaviour
anthropology
anti-capitalism
aquinas
archaeology
art
artificial intelligence
the baha'i faith
the beat generation
the bible
biodiversity
bioterror & biowarfare
the brain
british politics
the Buddha
cancer
censorship
christianity
civil liberties
classical music
climate change
cloning
the cold war
conservation
crimes against humanity
criminal psychology
critical thinking
the crusades
daoism
democracy
descartes
dewey
dyslexia
economics
energy

engineering
the english civil wars
the enlightenment
epistemology
ethics
the european union
evolution
evolutionary psychology
existentialism
fair trade
feminism
forensic science
french literature
the french revolution
genetics
global terrorism
hinduism
history
the history of medicine
history of science
homer
humanism
huxley
international relations
iran
islamic philosophy
the islamic veil
jazz
journalism
judaism
lacan
life in the universe
literary theory
machiavelli
mafia & organized crime
magic
marx
medieval philosophy
the middle east
modern slavery

NATO
the new testament
nietzsche
nineteenth-century art
the northern ireland conflict
nutrition
oil
opera
the palestine–israeli conflict
parapsychology
particle physics
paul
philosophy
philosophy of mind
philosophy of religion
philosophy of science
planet earth
postmodernism
psychology
quantum physics
the qur'an
racism
rawls
reductionism
religion
renaissance art
the roman empire
the russian revolution
shakespeare
shi'i islam
the small arms trade
stalin
sufism
the torah
the united nations
the victorians
volcanoes
the world trade organization
war
world war II

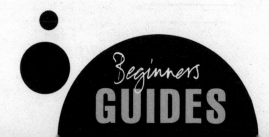

Cancer
A Beginner's Guide

Paul Scotting

Illustrated by Vanessa Appleby

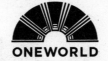

ONEWORLD

A Oneworld Book

First published by Oneworld Publications, 2010
This revised edition published by Oneworld Publications, 2017

ISBN 978-1- 78607-140-8
eISBN 978-1- 78607-141-5

Typeset by Jayvee, Trivandrum, India
Printed and bound in Great Britain by Clays Ltd, St Ives plc

Oneworld Publications
10 Bloomsbury Street
London WC1B 3SR
England

Contents

List of figures and tables   vii

Acknowledgements   viii

Second edition notes   x

Introduction   **1**

1   **A brief history of cancer**   **6**

Part 1: The selfish cell

2   **The circle of life**   17

3   **The immortal cell**   31

4   **Surviving and spreading**   39

Part 2: The enemy forces

5   **Mutation, mutation, mutation**   55

6   **Chemical carcinogens**   65

7   **Radiation**   77

8   **Catching cancer**   90

Part 3: Who gets cancer?

9 We are all different   101

10 Inheriting cancer   113

11 It shouldn't happen to children   124

Part 4: Winning the war

12 Attacking cancer   135

13 Prevention and cure: future
prospects   153

Appendix 1 DNA replication and
the cell cycle   181
Appendix 2 How DNA is repaired   190
Appendix 3 How infectious agents
cause cancer   192
Appendix 4 Inherited
predispositions to cancer   194

Glossary   199

Further reading   207

Index   212

List of figures and tables

Figure 1   Section from the Edwin Smith Papyrus   7

Figure 2   DNA bases and the structure of DNA   19

Figure 3   Gene expression   21

Figure 4   Inheritance of chromosomes during cell division   22

Figure 5   The cell cycle   24

Figure 6   Signalling pathways and the cell cycle   26

Figure 7   Metastasis of an epithelial tumour   43

Figure 8   The abnormal genome of cancers   57

Figure 9   Radiation-induced DNA damage   78

Figure 10   Variation in the incidence of malignant melanoma   80

Figure 11   The most common cancers in men and women in the UK   105

Figure 12   Worldwide incidence of prostate cancer   111

Figure 13   Inherited predisposition to cancer   115

Figure 14   Age distribution of cancers   124

Figure 15   Death rates from different classes of disease during the twentieth century   154

Figure 16   DNA replication   182

Figure 17   Regulation of the cell cycle   184

Table 1   The causes of cancer   60

Table 2   Main micro-organisms that play a role in cancer   90

Table 3   Familial cancer syndromes   118

Table 4   Avoidable causes of cancer in the UK   169

Acknowledgements

This book arose as a direct result of teaching a module in Cancer Genetics at the University of Nottingham with my colleagues Matt Loose and Jane Hewitt. I therefore owe a debt of gratitude to them, and to the many students who have gone through that course, for the pleasure and inspiration they have provided.

Having convinced myself that there was indeed a book to be written, my long-term colleague Ian Duce encouraged me to take it on, so he deserves a special mention along with my thanks to him, his wife Glenys and his daughter Carrie for reading an early draft.

Thanks to Andreas Leidenroth, Nicki Challenger, Annie Houldey, Helen Fielding and Trevor Ross-Gower, who all read the manuscript at various stages of completion and provided critical insights. My friend, Alison Symonds, merits special mention as my harshest critic, who, like my daughter, interpreted her task as teaching me English. Without them there would have been almost as many commas as there are words. Thanks to Susan Cleator and Carlo Palmeari for advice about breast cancer treatments and to Nick Bown for the images of chromosomes from normal and cancerous cells. I would like to make a special mention of Penny Howard (School of Nursing, Midwifery and Physiotherapy, Queens Medical School, Nottingham). Penny provided excellent advice on clinical matters and enthusiastic support for the project and she, above all others, contributed directly to the scientific content, especially in chapters 12 and 13.

I would like to thank Marsha Filion for so readily accepting this project for Oneworld Publications and for her reconstruction of my early efforts, and Mike Harpley for his help in the latter stages.

I must also thank my friends and colleagues in the Nottingham Children's Brain Tumour Research Centre. In particular, I thank David Walker and Jonathan Punt, for aiding and abetting my forays into the field of children's cancer research and Beth Coyle, a valued colleague with whom to discuss my ideas on children's cancer. Through them, I met Giorgio Perilongo, who convinced me that my ideas about cancer might be of some interest to others.

I would like to credit the charities – the Samantha Dickson Brain Tumour Trust, Ali's Dream, Charlie's Challenge and the Nottingham Children's Brain Tumour Research Centre – without whom I would never have been able to direct my fascination with cancer cells into real research. Also, thanks to Isabella Hildyard and her family for their support and encouragement in the early days of my research into children's brain tumours. Likewise, I would not have been able to carry out any of this work without the many students and researchers who have worked with me in my lab and those with whom I have collaborated.

I must especially thank my wife, Jane, and my kids, Oscar and Bertie, and above all Flo, who also read the second edition (some of it while awaiting the birth of her overdue first child, Fabian). Not only did they read various drafts of the book, but they also put up with endless 'here's another interesting fact about cancer' interjections at the dinner table.

Finally, cliché though it is, I want to thank my mum, Marion Scotting. Having read the manuscript, she described it as a 'page turner'. Biased though her opinion may be, I did not expect that it would achieve such an accolade, even from my own mother. The book is dedicated to her, because my success is her success, and so this book is as much her achievement as it is mine.

Second edition notes

Although the first edition of this book was well received, a number of readers felt that the sections discussing the biology of cells and DNA were rather difficult for the non-scientifically trained. In this edition I have therefore simplified these chapters, restricting their content to what is really essential to the understanding of later parts. The detail that has been removed is now available in the appendices for those who wish to understand the basic biology at a deeper level.

Many changes have been made in response to advances in our knowledge and understanding of cancer. Some of these are simply because time has elapsed. For example, the data on the survivors of the nuclear bomb attacks at Hiroshima and Nagasaki has now revealed a greater increase in the occurrence of solid cancers than was apparent at the time that the first edition was published. Numbers for the risk and survival for several of the cancer types have also been updated. Furthermore, in the past few years new information on the causes of lung cancer and the role of dietary components such as processed meats and alcohol in a wide range of cancers has come to light.

There have also been some significant changes in the available statistics for the risk of breast cancer in relation to hormone replacement therapies and screening. The section discussing the risks and benefits of breast cancer screening and the effects of using HRT have therefore been substantially updated.

It is never possible in such a fast-moving field to be up to date for long, but I have nevertheless provided information on the latest approaches to cancer therapies, especially those that aim to activate the immune system, which are currently at the forefront of new successes and have largely come to fruition since the publication of the first edition.

This edition ends with a broader consideration of what we can all do to avoid or reduce our risk of cancer. Much of this is very well known, such as avoiding tobacco smoke and excess UV light, etc. However, I also consider the potential role of other factors that might have a less pronounced impact on cancer risk, such as exercise or green tea.

Thanks to Shadi Doostdar of Oneworld for her helpful and thorough criticisms of this second edition. I would like to acknowledge all those who have posted reviews of the first edition of this book, especially those on the Macmillan website, since these have been a driving force for many of the changes in this edition.

Finally, this edition is dedicated to the hardworking nurses at Macmillan and, to put my money where my mouth is, all my royalties from the book's sales will go to that charity.

Introduction

Cancer is one of the most common life-threatening diseases of the modern world. Of all the potentially fatal diseases we are likely to encounter, cancer is second only to heart disease, killing one in four people in the West. We will all come into contact with it, either personally or as bystanders if friends and family are diagnosed with one of its different forms. And although many cancers are almost entirely curable with minimal therapy, this is not true of all of them. But do most of us really understand what cancer is?

We all know that cancer usually appears as a 'lump', an unwanted 'growth' called a 'tumour'. We know it can appear in almost any part of the body. We know that treatments for cancer can cause unpleasant side effects and that they do not always succeed in ridding us of the disease. However, most of us really have very little idea of the true nature of cancer. A clear insight into the biology of cancer is essential for scientists and clinicians, but I believe we can all deal better with the consequences of cancer if we really understand what it is.

For many, cancer is seen as an alien intent on our destruction. It grows inside our bodies, eventually overwhelming our life-support systems. Its purpose is to destroy us, for its own benefit. While this would be a good description of many diseases, it is not a fair portrait of cancer. The drug-resistant 'superbug' Methicillin-Resistant Staphylococcus Aureus (MRSA), which lurks in our hospital wards, is indeed such an alien invader. It does attempt to destroy us for its own benefit and moves on to a new host at the first opportunity. Viruses, for example the Human Immunodeficiency Virus, HIV (which causes AIDS), are even more sinister in their behaviour. They invade us, enter the body's cells and use the cells' own machinery to provide the building blocks they need to replicate themselves before they leave the body and spread to another victim. Their host's demise is of no consequence to them; viruses have evolved to feed upon us for the good of their own kind.

Cancer is different. It arises from our own flesh and blood. Our bodies are composed of billions of individual cells, organized into tissues such as bone, muscle or skin, that together build our functional organs. The cells of a cancer, which can increase in number to a point when we are eventually left unable to fight them off, are our own cells. Despite its reputation as an aggressive 'being', a cancer gains no benefit from its host's eventual downfall. Cancer cells don't survive when we give up the fight; they do not move on to a new host. They are part of us and they die with us.

Cancers normally arise when, due to damage – mutations – to its genes, just one cell escapes the many controls that make it behave correctly. It is as if a person develops a fatal flaw in their ability to behave in the way their society requires and instead causes mayhem in the community. You might ask 'What is acceptable behaviour for a cell?' As with people, this depends very much on when and where you ask the question. Behaviour that is acceptable in a young, developing child may be far from acceptable in an adult. It's the same for cells: the cells in a baby abide by rather different rules from those in an adult. It's absolutely fine for the cells of a baby's growing bones to increase rapidly in number, but this behaviour would be disastrous in the limbs of an adult. Similarly, it is essential for cells in a baby's developing nervous system to migrate through the body as it grows, but we certainly don't want this to happen once the body is fully formed. Even within a specific tissue, it is fine for some cells to increase in number rapidly, but totally unacceptable for others. These are exactly the sorts of behaviours that go wrong in cancer.

Cancer is the result of cells acquiring many abnormalities in their behaviour. Among these abnormalities are the abilities to produce more cells in an uncontrolled manner, to become immortal and avoid any urge to die and to spread throughout the body. Cells that will become a cancer make these changes gradually, overcoming the many safeguards that normally ensure cells stay on the straight and narrow. When only some of these behaviours have been acquired – for example, uncontrolled growth and immortality – the cells can form an abnormal tissue mass, a *benign* tumour, which can readily be removed and cured. The gradual change from normal cell, to benign tumour to a cancer that can be described as malignant ('showing intense ill will') is called *tumour progression*. I will talk more about tumour progression in Parts 1 and 2.

Even those who spend their lives treating or studying cancer often have only a superficial understanding of aspects of cancer distant from their specialist interest. One reason for this surprising lack of knowledge, given the prevalence of cancer, is that there is no book specifically designed to explain the many issues related to cancer in a clear and straightforward way. This is why I decided to write this book. I will describe what goes wrong in the rogue cells we call cancer, what causes these defects and how scientists and doctors are attempting to remove the wayward cells from our bodies.

This book is aimed primarily at people who want to better understand what cancer is, how we can try to avoid it and how we can treat it. The topics I will cover range from the basic biology of the cell and how this is disrupted in cancer to the underlying mechanisms of cancer therapies and the latest research and successes in developing more effective and less toxic treatments for cancer.

The study of cancer has revealed some of the beauty of how cells work. It is my interest in the intricacies of how things work that drives me as much as the desire to solve the problem of cancer. Indeed, a cell holds as much fascination for me as the mechanisms of the whole organism. John Ruskin put this better than I could, although in a rather different context:

> For a stone, when it is examined, will be found a mountain in miniature. The fineness of Nature's work is so great, that into a single block, a foot or two in diameter, she can compress as many changes of form and structure, on a small scale, as she needs for her mountains on a large one.[*]

At the start of the twentieth century, cancer had been studied for many hundreds of years, but we had almost no understanding of its nature. Paul Kraske (1851–1930), a German surgeon, said 'We do not know any more about cancer than our grandfathers did.' I think it is safe to say that we now know a great deal more than did our grandfathers, or even our fathers. There can be little doubt that the late twentieth century saw unprecedented progress in cancer research and understanding and much-improved therapies. Since the early 1970s, the proportion of people in England and Wales surviving cancer for 10 years or more has more than doubled. For some cancers the improvement has been even more dramatic. Leukaemias are the most notable, with 10-year survival increasing almost sevenfold (6.8% to 46% between 1971 and 2011). An even greater rate of improvement is likely in the early decades of the twenty-first century. I hope that by reading this book you will not only develop a better understanding of what cancer is, why cancer happens and how treatments work, but also a confidence that things are now better than ever before and will get better still.

Whether you are simply interested in cancer as a fascinating biological phenomenon, or you have a personal reason, such as

---

[*] From John Ruskin's *Frondes Agrestes: Readings in Modern Painters*, Section VI. First published in 1875

you or someone you know being affected by cancer, I hope you will find the book both accessible and informative. This is not, however, a book that aims to advise you on how to cope or live with cancer – there are very many books available that purport to serve that purpose. I have also kept in mind those whom I have taught over the years. I hope this book will be a primer for undergraduates studying nursing, medicine and the biological sciences and, in addition, provide the broad overview of many aspects of cancer and its biology that such courses tend to lack due to the time constraints of individual curricula. Hence, I hope that undergraduates and older school students will find this book a valuable addition to their more specialized reading, providing a comprehensive review of the various issues that we must consider when studying the disease we call 'cancer'. To this end, I have included appendices covering some of the more complex issues in more detail, for those who want more depth of coverage.

1
A brief history of cancer

The damage that causes cancer is usually due to toxic agents – carcinogens – including chemicals and radiation, which alter our genes. Cancer is the final result of the multiple damaging events these carcinogens cause in a single cell.

There are two opposing views of the history of cancer. One is that cancer has always been here: as long as there has been life, there has been cancer. The opposing view is that because many of the carcinogens that cause cancer have only become widespread in the environment since the Industrial Revolution in the eighteenth century, cancer is a disease of the modern age. It seems there is some truth in both views. For humans – and other animals – cancer has always been with us, but many of the more common cancers have only become prevalent in the last few hundred years.

The problem with trying to determine the extent to which cancers were present in earlier centuries is that before the late seventeenth century the way in which patients were examined would not have revealed most types of cancer. Also, the term 'cancer' was applied to a wide range of growths, many of which would not now be classified as cancers. The earliest recorded descriptions of cancer come from Ancient Egypt. One document, known as the Edwin Smith Papyrus, written between 3000 and 1500 BCE, is regarded as one of the oldest medical records. Edwin Smith, an American, was described as 'an adventurer, a money lender and a dealer of antiquities'. In 1862, he bought the manuscript from a dealer in the city of Luxor in Egypt and, although he recognized its importance, a full translation (by James Henry Breasted) was not published until 1930, some years after Smith's death. The manuscript's descriptions of 48 patients include several suffering from a disease that would now be recognized as breast cancer.

There is also some archaeological evidence to suggest that humans suffered from cancer in the Bronze Age (1900–1600 BCE). Strikingly, these archaeological examples are often of bone cancer, which is now relatively rare. However, we should beware of jumping to conclusions. Such observations do not imply that bone cancer used to be more common; the remains

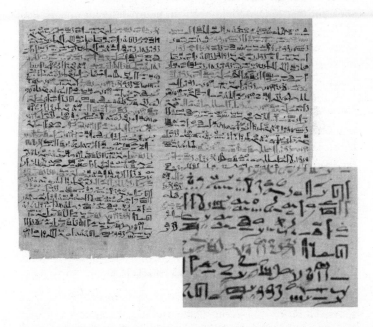

Figure 1 Section from the Edwin Smith Papyrus, which describes 48 patients, including some with breast cancer

often include little other than bone, so there is not much scope to find clear evidence of any other kind of cancer. From Ancient Greece to Roman times, the majority of descriptions of cancer refer to the female breast. Aulus Cornelius Celsus (30 BCE–38 CE), commented on the relatively limited distribution of cancers diagnosed at this time, stating that cancer 'occurs mainly in the upper structures about the face, nose, ears and lips and female breasts'. While most cases described were cancers of the breast, cancers of the uterus and digestive tract were also known. Despite this, even Galen, whose descriptions of cancer provided the basic reference for clinicians from their time of writing (131–203 CE) until the late eighteenth century, appeared to be largely unaware of cancers of the internal organs. By the seventh century, it was apparent that cancer could occur in many different organs. Paul of Aegina (625–690 CE) correctly noted that cancer arises in every part of the body, even the eyes and the uterus, but he went on to suggest that 'it is especially common in women's breasts because they are lax and quickly take up the coarsest matter'!

Little progress in understanding was then made over the next 1,000 years. One of the most useful observations, providing an indication of the thinking of the time, was made by Hieronymus Fabricius (1537–1619) of Padua, Italy, who stated that 'the lung, the liver and the soft structures can scarcely become cancerous'. Despite the identification of cancers in a wide range of organs, they were still rare in comparison to cancers of the breast and uterus, the reasons for which will be discussed shortly.

Cancer since the Renaissance

The eighteenth century saw a development in medicine that at last allowed a major leap in our understanding of cancer: the advent of autopsy (in which the body is dissected to determine the cause of death). Giovanni Battista Morgagni, Professor of Anatomy of the University of Padua, published *The seats and causes of diseases investigated by anatomy*, a well-described procedure for autopsy. Morgagni was a powerful intellectual force from the time of his graduation at the age of 19, with a degree in medicine and philosophy, to his 79th year, when he published his seminal work. He also found time to father 15 children and establish himself as a renowned archaeologist. Morgagni was widely respected for his works on anatomy, which provided accurate anatomical explanations for the features seen in disease, as opposed to the speculations, based on little real evidence, that were typical of earlier centuries. He spent his life recounting the outcomes of his many autopsies and providing anatomical descriptions of the human organs, both healthy and diseased, including cancers.

From the eighteenth century onwards, although descriptions of many different cancers appeared, including those of the face, rectum, stomach, penis and the female genitalia, descriptions of breast cancer still outnumbered all other types. It seems that those cancers that we now know to be linked to modern carcinogens were comparatively rare before the twentieth century, while others such as breast cancer (which appears to be more intrinsic to the body, with a strong genetic predisposition, chapter 9, p. 104–107; chapter 10, p. 120–121) were more common.

The number of carcinogen-driven cancers has fluctuated dramatically depending on exposure to particular agents. Lung cancer provides one very striking example of this. In 1878, a study of all cancers seen at autopsy in the Institute of Pathology of the University of Dresden in Germany identified only 1% as malignant lung tumours. By 1918, when the smoking of rolled cigarettes had become widespread, the percentage had risen to almost 10% and by 1927 to more than 14%, a number that remains similar in most Western countries today.

In some cases, cancers caused by occupational carcinogens appeared early in modern history and, thanks to the insight of clinicians of the time, were identified and dealt with. One example was a condition known to chimney sweeps as 'soot-wart'. This was in fact cancer of the scrotum, first described by Percivall Pott in 1775. It soon became clear that this cancer was due to soot (now known to contain powerful carcinogens) becoming lodged in the 'moist rugae' of the scrotum. By the late nineteenth century, guidance from the chimney sweeps guild of Denmark for sweeps to take daily baths had resulted in great improvements, as was noted in a report in the *British Medical Journal* in 1892, entitled 'Why foreign sweeps do not suffer from scrotal cancer'. This was a reflection of the rather less hygienic habits of British sweeps, who unfortunately continued to develop this cancer for some time. Interestingly, there was a clear recognition of the ability of cancer to spread within the body. Percivall Pott writes:

> If there be any chance of putting a stop to or preventing this mischief, it must be by the immediate removal of the part affected; I mean that part of the scrotum where the sore is; for if it be suffered to remain until the virus has seized the testicle, it is generally too late even for castration. I have many times made the experiment; but though the sores, after such operation, have, in some instances, healed kindly and the patients have gone from the hospital seemingly well, yet, in the space of a few months, it has generally happened, that they have returned, either with the same disease in the other testicle or in the glands of the groin, to with such wan complexions, such pale leaden countenances, such a total loss of strength and such frequent and acute internal pains, as have sufficiently proved a diseased state of some of the viscera and which have soon been followed by a painful death.

Throughout the 1800s, many, like Percivall Pott, continued to believe that cancer was caused by an infectious agent. This belief was partly due to a phenomenon termed cancer *à deux*, in which married couples were noted both to develop cancer. We now understand that there are two good explanations for cancer *à deux*. First, the cancers concerned were often of the genitalia (such as in the cervix or penis), which are now known to be unusual cancers in which viral infection plays a significant role (see chapter 9), and, second, many couples would both have been exposed to the same carcinogens in their environment. The fact that cancer could be transferred from one region of the body to another, or to experimental animals, was also generally taken as evidence of an infectious cause rather than the ability of cancer cells to spread.

Finally, by the beginning of the twentieth century, developments in the detailed study of diseased tissue meant that the true composition of cancer, derived from our own cells, was clearly established.

A disease of the modern age?

Although it is clear that cancer has been observed since records began, it is also evident that cancer became increasingly common during the twentieth century. One explanation for this increase is that improvements in quality of life and healthcare have resulted in our living to a greater age. Before about 1800, average life expectancy was fairly stable at around 40 to 45 years; since most cancers do not occur until we reach old age, there was much less opportunity for it to occur in centuries gone by. In short, other diseases got us before cancer had a chance. Of course, even in ancient history, some people did live to old age, so there was still the opportunity for carcinogenic damage to accumulate over many decades. A range of cancers was seen, but their numbers seem to have been far fewer than we see now. In the nineteenth and twentieth centuries, life expectancy doubled in many parts of the world to the 70 or 80 years we can now anticipate in developed countries such as the UK. Our bodies now provide the necessary time for cancer to develop and so it has become one of the most common causes of death.

Another explanation for the recent increase in cancer numbers is that exposure to most common carcinogens is relatively new. For example, sunlight has become a greater cause of skin cancer now than it was many years ago. This is because sudden or strong exposure to ultraviolet light contributes to skin cancer in those who are not normally exposed to it. In years gone by, exposure to the sun was continuous for those living and working outdoors. Pigment therefore accumulated, which protected the skin cells from the effects of ultraviolet light. Also, fashion and the rules of social decency meant that people in the northern hemisphere covered up most of their skin when outdoors – the phenomenon of sunbathing only became popular after the 1920s. It seems that this change in our habits has given rise to one of the most dramatic increases in cancer occurrence: incidence of malignant skin cancer has increased more than fourfold in the UK since the mid-1970s. Because it usually takes 15 to 30 years for a cancer to appear after the initial exposure to a carcinogen, this increase possibly reflects a change in habits dating back to the 1950s and 1960s, a period that coincided with an upsurge in foreign travel and a significant decline in the amount of clothing worn when in the sun. Our awareness of the risks of sunburn does now seem to be affecting our behaviour; the sunblocks we use are much more effective and we pay more attention to protecting children from sunburn. We can only hope that this will lead to a decrease in the incidence of aggressive skin cancer over the next 25 years.

But what about breast cancer, which, above all other cancers, is frequently described in historical texts? Although breast cancer has always been one of the most common cancers, it seems probable that it too was significantly less common in earlier times than it is now. As I will discuss in chapter 9, early childbirth and prolonged breastfeeding both protect against breast cancer. In economically developed countries, the nature of families and pregnancy changed dramatically in the nineteenth and twentieth centuries. In the USA, average family size fell from 7 children in the early 1800s to 3.5 children by 1900 and, as the twentieth century progressed, to the current level of around 2. The trend towards smaller family size and later first pregnancies means that women have largely lost the benefits of these protective factors against breast cancer.

Although it seems that breast cancer, in particular, is likely to have been prevalent in historic times, by the beginning of the twentieth century the range of cancers with which we are now familiar was evident and scientists and clinicians had begun to view cancer as our own cells gone wrong. However, an almost total lack of understanding meant surgical removal of tumours was the only means of treatment. Not until the advent of recombinant DNA technology ('gene cloning'), in the late 1970s, did we at last have the means to gain real insights into cancers' biology; insights that, at last, have heralded the advent of new therapies, with the promise of more on the horizon.

Summary

It appears that cancer has always been associated with human life. However, it is most prevalent in older people and it is more common following exposure to environmental carcinogens that damage DNA. Cancer has therefore become a much more prevalent problem in most countries since the industrial age, when life expectancies and exposure to carcinogens both increased. We now understand what most of these causes are, so public health messages and public policy could begin to protect us from their effects. Unfortunately, it is not always easy to get the public to heed these messages.

Part 1
The selfish cell

2
The circle of life

To understand how one of our own cells can become so antisocial as to become cancerous, we need to understand some basic features of normal cell function. One of the most important aspects of a cell's behaviour is whether or not it divides, because this is often the first thing to go wrong in cancer.

How cells divide

As our bodies grow, our cells divide many times to produce the millions of cells that make up each of our organs. While cells are dividing, they are referred to as *undifferentiated*, meaning that they have few of the specific features of a useful, grown-up cell. Some of those cells then stop dividing and undergo the process of *differentiation*, in which the cell changes dramatically to acquire the features it needs to contribute to the functions of its organ: for example, neurons producing neurotransmitters in the brain, hair cells in the skin or acid-secreting cells in the gut. Once our organs are fully formed, most of their cells are differentiated and function as active members of the tissue community, carrying out the complex tasks required of them.

Cells that are no longer dividing need regular replacement. Such differentiated cells have a limited life-span and are doomed to die, with the notable exception of the neurons of the brain (which are almost entirely produced by the end of our first year of life and must last us a lifetime). In most organs, cells die in days or weeks and must be replenished. For this reason, even as adults, our tissues still contain some dividing cells. However, these cells are not cancerous, because they stop dividing at the appropriate time. Many safeguards exist, ready to block cells from division except where it is expressly desired for the growth and function of the body. It is therefore surprising that cells ever manage to overcome these controls and proliferate to cause cancer – but they do. Not only is endless proliferation the most obvious feature of cancerous cells, it is often the first mistake these cells make. As will become clear, this is the first of many mistakes.

How do cells divide? We often refer to one cell as the 'mother cell' and to the cells that are produced by its division as 'daughter cells'. The mother cell grows rapidly, getting fatter and fatter over the space of hours, and then splits in two, each half becoming a daughter cell. However, they aren't like animal mothers and daughters, for the mother no longer exists after division; it is replaced by the two daughter cells, each of which inherits about half the entire being of the mother. So, division requires the mother cell to double all its various contents and separate them evenly into the two daughter cells. This represents a remarkable achievement in only a few hours.

The daughter cells might stop and differentiate into mature, fully functional cells or they might become mother cells themselves and divide again, thus going back to the beginning of the doubling process. As far as cancer is concerned, the most critical feature of cell division is the correct replication of the DNA genome, since it is damage to our genes that is at the root of almost all cancers. Each daughter cell must inherit a perfect copy of the mother's genes.

THE STRUCTURE OF DNA

Our genes are part of our DNA (*deoxyribonucleic acid*), which exists as long, intertwined, paired strands held together by so-called hydrogen bonds. In every human cell, an identical copy of that DNA, our *genome*, is shared between 23 separate pairs of chromosomes – one set of 23 inherited from each parent. The strands have a uniform backbone made up of repeated units of a sugar molecule, deoxyribose, and to each deoxyribose unit is attached a *base*. Together, the deoxyribose and base make up a *nucleotide*; DNA strands are made up of chains of nucleotides, linked by phosphate groups.

There are just four different bases, guanine, cytosine, adenine and thymine (usually abbreviated to G, C, A and T), but their precise order in the DNA strand forms a simple code, crucial to the function of DNA.

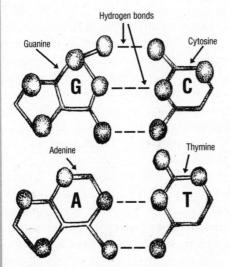

Formation of hydrogen bonds between Gs and Cs, and between As and Ts, allows nucleotides in the DNA strands to pair.

Figure 2   DNA bases and the structure of DNA

How genes work

Our genes are the parts of our DNA that act as blueprints, instructing the cell which proteins it should make. Proteins have many different functions: some give the cell its shape or its ability to move, others are enzymes that allow other chemicals to be made or food to be digested and used for energy. Many act as signals, either inside the cell or outside it, released to pass messages to other cells. Almost every functional aspect of a cell's life is governed by specific proteins, all of which are there only as a result of a gene being switched on so its code can be interpreted or 'expressed'. The particular genes that are expressed (that is, the mix of genes that are on or off), and therefore the proteins that a cell contains, determine what type of cell it is and how it behaves.

The first step in this process of gene expression is *transcription*, when the precise sequence of the DNA bases (A, G, C and T) is copied into a similar chain of bases, RNA (*ribonucleic acid*), which has a slightly different chemical backbone from DNA. The RNA escapes from the nucleus into the main body of the cell, the soup of chemicals called the *cytoplasm*. Once in the cytoplasm, the RNA reaches the *ribosomes*, highly complex molecular machines that use the RNA as a template for the production of proteins. Each group of three bases, a *codon*, in the RNA represents a code (identical to the code in the gene from which it was copied) that determines which sub-unit, called an amino acid, will be added to the growing protein. As the RNA is spooled through the ribosome, the growing protein chain of amino acids is synthesized. Although each cell in our bodies contains identical genes, the particular set of genes expressed by the cell determines its particular protein content.

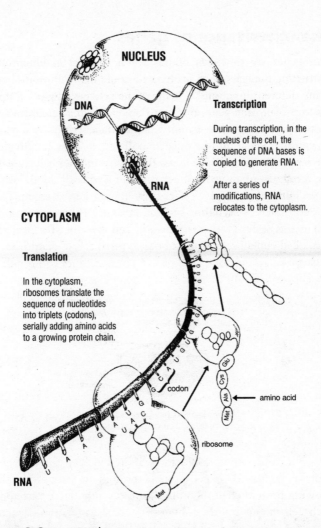

Figure 3 Gene expression
Genes are 'transcribed' into RNA, which is then exported into the cyto-plasm where it is 'translated' into proteins by the ribosomes.

The inheritance of genes

There are two senses in which our genes are inherited. We inherit a complete set of genes on one set of 23 chromosomes from each of our parents. We therefore have two slightly different copies of each gene, one from our father and one from our mother, and these give us our unique characteristics, a bit like our mother and a bit like our father. Then, as each cell divides, the new cells inherit their genes from their mother cell. One of the most important goals of cell division is to replicate the cell's DNA and leave a single perfect copy in each new daughter cell: this way, each cell acquires exactly the same DNA as every other cell in the body. From the very first cell division of a fertilized egg, all dividing cells in our bodies, for the rest of our lives, must make a new copy of those 46 chromosomes to provide a

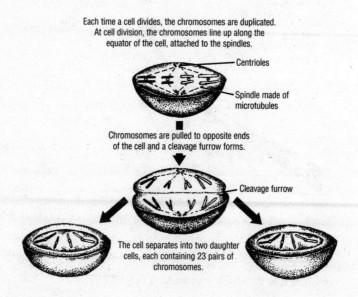

Each time a cell divides, the chromosomes are duplicated. At cell division, the chromosomes line up along the equator of the cell, attached to the spindles.

Centrioles

Spindle made of microtubules

Chromosomes are pulled to opposite ends of the cell and a cleavage furrow forms.

Cleavage furrow

The cell separates into two daughter cells, each containing 23 pairs of chromosomes.

Figure 4 Inheritance of chromosomes during cell division

full complement for each of the daughter cells that are formed. Once the new chromosomes are complete, the cell machinery pulls one of each identical pair towards each end of the original cell before it finally divides in two.

The cell cycle

To divide successfully, the replication of our genome must be precisely co-ordinated with all the other events needed for the cell to duplicate its contents and split in two. The tightly regulated process from single cell to two new cells is called the *cell cycle*.

The machinery of the cell cycle is made up of hundreds or thousands of different molecules, most of which are distributed semi-randomly within the cell. Despite this, there are many ways in which the key components are linked, so that they behave in an integrated way. The resulting system can be thought of like the parts of a motor or a clock, intimately locked together. Through these links, synthesis of the DNA and the other cell components, such as the cell membrane, is co-ordinated. The subsequent separation of the newly made chromosomes and the division of the cell into two daughter cells then happens in a beautifully synchronized fashion, ensuring that each new cell acquires its full complement of 23 chromosome pairs.

With respect to cancer, the key events in the cell cycle are the replication of the chromosomes to make perfect duplicate copies and the separation of the two copies, one into each of the two daughter cells. These processes are policed by proteins that make sure each step only happens when it should and that the cell does not continue through the cell cycle if errors occur. To begin DNA replication, the cell cycle must pass a stage called the *restriction point*. This point is only passed if the cell receives signals from outside the cell that tell it that now is the right time and place to replicate. These signals are usually proteins, often so-called growth factors, made by other cells. The signalling cells may be nearby, or some distance away so the signal protein has to travel in the blood. Once the restriction point is passed, the cell is no longer sensitive to influences from outside the cell.

In addition, there are several checkpoints in the cell cycle at which proteins within the cell, referred to as gatekeepers, can sense if there is a problem, such as an error in replication of the DNA or the chromosomes not being ready to be pulled apart. If the gatekeepers are activated, they will block the cell cycle so that repair systems (sometimes referred to as caretakers) can be activated and the error corrected before the cycle restarts. At each of the checkpoints there are key proteins that act as the final switch turning the cell cycle on or off. For the restriction

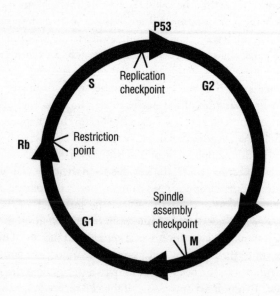

Figure 5 The cell cycle

point (which links the cell cycle to the outside world of the cell) the protein Rb (named after the cancer with which it is most strongly associated, retinoblastoma) is the key switch. For the checkpoints that sense errors within the cell, the key switch is a protein called P53, which, among other functions, can pause the cell cycle while the DNA is repaired.

The precise control of the cell cycle is a complex, beautiful and intensely researched area. For those who would like to read more about it, I discuss this aspect of cell biology in more detail in Appendix 1.

Growth signals

Cells are continuously subject to a battery of external signals that regulate almost all aspects of their behaviour. To be sensitive to these signals, they carry a vast array of receptor proteins for these signals on their surface. The activation of many of these receptors determines whether or not a cell will divide. Cells respond to these signals by changing the genes that they switch on and off to produce the key proteins needed for that cell's behaviour. When the signal affects the cell cycle, the outcome determines whether the cell passes the restriction point. This is achieved by switching the Rb protein on or off, so the cell cycle is inhibited or activated respectively.

What goes wrong?

The genes that can cause the initiation of cancer when they are mutated or de-regulated fall into one of two classes. The bad guys, which promote cancer development if they are activated, are called *oncogenes*. The good guys, which normally protect the cell from these behaviours, and must be inactivated in cancer cells, are termed *tumour suppressors*. Many cancers involve both

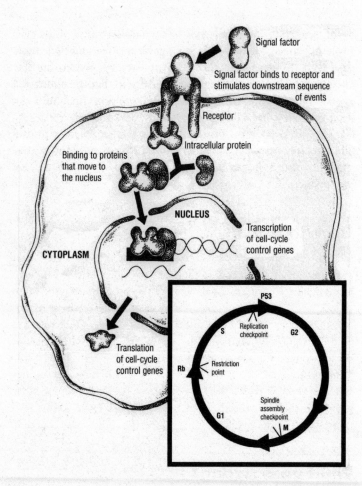

Figure 6 Signalling pathways and the cell cycle

the activation of oncogenes and the inactivation of tumour suppressors. In addition, later mutations affect genes that contribute to the progression of the tumour, such as their ability to spread throughout the body.

Activation of almost any step in a signalling pathway can play a role in cancer. However, it is a significant over-simplification to suggest that each step in these pathways acts to activate the next; many steps actually inhibit the next step, but the end result can still be activation of the final gene expression. Imagine a car on a hill: you can make it go by putting your foot on the accelerator or you can make it go by releasing the handbrake that was inhibiting the rotation of the wheels. Similarly, mutations that affect the signalling pathways take effect either by activating an oncogene (accelerator) that promotes cancerous growth or by inactivating a tumour suppressor (brake) that inhibits it. Just like the car, releasing the brake is pretty much essential to get the cancer moving. So it is that at least one tumour suppressor gene is found to be mutated in almost all cancers.

One way or another, disruption of at least one component of the signalling pathways that tell cells whether or not to proliferate is seen in almost all cancers. Once cells begin to proliferate excessively, the chances of this developing into a full-blown cancer are substantially increased, because mutations occur through the process of DNA synthesis. The more DNA synthesis there is, the greater the chances of further damaging mutations occurring. This is why a highly proliferative cell population has an increased probability of incurring a mutation, which could then trigger the next step towards cancer.

Damage to gatekeepers and caretakers

If any of the signalling events above become disrupted by mutation of any component, uncontrolled proliferation might ensue. However, even then, this alone would not give rise to cancer. A group of cells simply over-proliferating would form only a small benign tumour. For a benign tumour to progress to a fully malignant cancer, many more processes must be disrupted. This requires many mutations – most scientists would accept six as a reasonable estimate.

The frequency of mutation resulting accidentally from the imperfect nature of DNA replication is about one mutation in any given gene in every 10,000,000 (10^7) cell divisions. (Mathematically, for ease of writing, large numbers are often written as 10^x; so 10^7 means 1 followed by 7 zeros.) This means that mutation of any six specific genes in the same single cell would only occur about once in every 10^{42} cells. This equates to one cell in every 10^{29} people; with fewer than ten billion (10^{10}) people on Earth, this would mean cancer would never occur. It is clear, then, that mutations must occur much more often than this background error rate for cancer to be seen so often in the human population. This is due to the effects of carcinogens (discussed in detail in chapters 6 and 7) and the cells themselves becoming more prone to mutation.

Cancer arises because the proteins that normally ensure the proper repair of DNA damage, themselves become defective due to mutations in the genes that code for those proteins. This makes the cells even more prone to mutations and so causes an increase in the rate that mutations are acquired. Mutations that affect this machinery are generally early events in cancer cells, leading to cells acquiring the additional mutations necessary to develop into full-blown cancer. Only when the mutation rate increases can enough events be disrupted within a single cell within our lifetime for cancer to arise. One protein appears to be so important in the link between DNA repair and cell cycle control that it is mutated in most types of cancer. This protein is P53. Depending on the type of cancer in question, the P53 gene is mutated in 30–50% of cases. The consequence of such mutations is that the cell cycle is no longer properly regulated and cells can continue to divide without having to wait for DNA damage to be repaired. This causes cells to replicate damaged DNA, each generation of daughter cells acquiring more and more mutations. This state is referred to as a *mutator phenotype* – in other words, a state in which the proteins that police the cell cycle and the DNA repair machinery are themselves so defective that the cell rapidly accumulates many more mutations (by the time they are diagnosed, cancer cells can carry tens of thousands of mutations). In some of those cells, the result could be damage to key processes necessary for the cell to remain viable and so it dies, but in others it could be damage to the very genes needed to protect the cell from the behaviours that are characteristic of cancer, so cancer will ensue.

As cancers progress, the increasing number of mutations affect other cell systems. One of the most important is the spindle checkpoint, which regulates the separation of the chromosomes into the two daughter cells. This should happen only when their replication and alignment is perfect. When this checkpoint is faulty, even more profound damage results, as the spindle pulls the chromosomes apart even when some chromosomes aren't properly attached. This results in different numbers of chromosomes being inherited by each daughter cell.

Despite the many levels of control of the cell cycle, cancer cells can circumvent them in many different ways. Cancer cells are like factories in which the machine operators, the regulators overseeing the machine operators and sometimes the machine itself are malfunctioning. Fortunately, another feature of cells protects us from the growth that would otherwise arise when such damage has occurred. All the potentially cancerous events that lead to an increased drive to proliferate come to nothing if the cells die. Unfortunately, as we will see in the next chapter, the normal version of P53 plays a central role in protecting the cell from cancer, by assisting the cells to die if any damage cannot be repaired. This helps to explain why its function is disrupted in so many cancers; when they are damaged, the cells not only proliferate excessively, but they also survive when they should die.

Summary

Our bodies contain large pools of dividing cells throughout our lives and it is these cells that provide the opportunity for cancer to develop. All dividing cells must replicate their DNA and it is during DNA replication that errors can occur, resulting in mutations. The nature of cell division means that mutations are passed on through the generations of those dividing cells. The change of a single base, A, G, C or T, in just one gene, can cause cancer to start if that mutation activates an oncogene or inactivates a tumour suppressor gene.

3
The immortal cell

As we progress through life, the continued production of cells is a necessary feature in the maintenance of most of our organs. This is largely because the mature cells that are the components of our tissues have a relatively limited lifespan and simply wear out. However, in addition to wear and tear, our cells can also undergo a kind of intentional cell death. This process has become known as *programmed cell death*, the best-studied form of which is *apoptosis* (from the Greek for 'falling off'). This process of active cell suicide is not the only mechanism by which cells are lost. Most cells of most animals also have a built-in ageing process; after a finite number of cell divisions, they cannot continue to proliferate so they simply stop dividing. This process, *senescence*, is believed to play a central role in the ageing process of our bodies as a whole.

For cells to become cancerous, they must overcome both the self-destructive tendencies of apoptosis and the natural ageing process of senescence, so they can carry on living and dividing despite having acquired potentially devastating genome damage. Unfortunately, the catastrophic mutational events in a cancer cell not only cause them to divide uncontrollably, but also leave them unable to die. They are likely to attempt to die, but, like a super-human immortal being, they can never achieve it. In the absence of a successful treatment, they are doomed to grow and grow.

Senescence

The reason cells are not normally immortal is due to the gradual decay of chromosomes every time a cell divides. Each time these massive strands of DNA are copied, the ends get missed, and the chromosome becomes a little shorter. As protection from this potential damage, the ends of the chromosomes do not carry any information critical to the cells' function. Instead, they are made up of short repeated DNA sequences called *telomeres*. The gradual shortening of the ends of our chromosomes has little impact on the cell's behaviour; it simply reduces the number of telomere repeats. However, there does come a point (named the Hayflick limit, after its discoverer), on average after about 50 cell divisions, at which the telomere DNA becomes too short and so the more important genes become vulnerable. Cells can sense when this point is reached. When the cell is young, the telomeres appear to loop around, hiding the exposed end of the chromosome, which would otherwise look just like a broken DNA end. When the number of telomeres drops below a critical level, the machinery of the cell recognizes the ends as DNA breaks. One consequence is that the P53 and Rb systems (which control cell division) are activated

EVERLASTING ANIMALS

Although it seems likely that telomere shortening may have in part evolved to protect our cells from readily becoming cancerous, it isn't seen in all animals.

Some animals, such as crocodiles, lobsters and turtles, express telomerase (the enzyme that causes the addition of telomeres at the ends of the chromosomes) throughout their bodies and throughout their lives. Interestingly, these animals appear to lack a finite lifespan and tend not to be limited by body size. It seems that such animals do not age like we do but eventually die from disease or other vagaries of living in the wild. Why they have evolved differently is unclear. They are certainly not renowned for their high incidence of tumours, so presumably they avoid cancer by other means.

and trigger the cell to enter the state of senescence. Instead of beginning DNA replication, the cell leaves the cell cycle and adopts this inert state of suspended animation. The cell does not die, or differentiate into a fully functional, mature cell; it is simply, irreversibly, stopped.

Clearly, this phenomenon, in which cells stop proliferating after a given number of cell divisions, has the potential to limit the growth of a tumour. The tumour might grow for a while, but there would come a time when the cells reached senescence and stopped dividing. We would see the spontaneous arrest of the tumour growth, and that is precisely what we do see. This is one reason why benign tumours do not become cancers. Most of us have many benign tumours, the most obvious of which are moles, pigmented skin cells that have acquired some genetic damage, leading to unregulated proliferation. However, the cells of moles do not escape senescence so, after they have continued to divide for a short while, they simply stop growing. Unfortunately, if just one more mutation allows these cells to overcome senescence, they are well on their way to becoming potentially fatal skin cancer – malignant melanoma. Fortunately the vast majority of moles never make that transition and are forever limited by senescence.

How do cancer cells avoid this natural ageing process? A clue comes from laboratory experiments on growing cells. When cells grown in a plastic dish in the laboratory reach the point when senescence might occur, a very small number acquire the ability to circumvent this fate (for example by mutation of P53) and continue to divide, their chromosomes getting ever shorter. When the number of telomeres is reduced even further, the cells reach a point when the chromosomes become highly unstable. The cell sees the ends of the chromosome as DNA breaks and tries to repair them by joining them to other broken ends, jumbling the sequences between different chromosomes, so called *recombination*. When cells reach this stage, the typical response is cell death via apoptosis. However, a very few cells, probably fewer than one in a million, manage to survive and continue to divide, able to grow on indefinitely, becoming immortal. When we look to determine what has changed in these rare immortal cells, we find they have activated an enzyme, *telomerase*, which can initiate the renewal of the telomeres.

Given that cancer cells must divide many more times than normal cells, some means of avoiding senescence is essential. Activating telomerase appears to be an almost universal event in cancer; over 90% of tumours show reactivated telomerase activity. It seems that a cancer cell will usually reach a point at which its chromosomes become subject to rearrangements due to telomere loss. The cancer cell breaches this barrier by reactivating telomerase so that it continues to divide. The result is an immortal cell, with substantial genetic damage.

Apoptosis

Not only do cells stop dividing as they age, but they also have the ability to kill themselves. Cell suicide is not only frequent – it is expected. Like Captain Lawrence Oates who famously 'just went outside' during the Scott expedition to the South Pole in 1912, some cells take their own lives apparently for the good of their comrades.

There are two main reasons why cells choose to die through programmed cell death (*apoptosis*). As the body develops in the womb, its structures are not made according to a carefully laid-out plan, in which each part is precisely placed until, as in a jigsaw puzzle, the last piece makes them complete. Rather, they are formed like a fine sculpture made from clay, in which the raw material is moulded into an approximate form, which the artist then carefully trims and cuts to make the shape perfect. Hands and feet first form as crude paddles and then, by carefully regimented mass suicide, cells are removed, leaving individual digits behind. In a similar but less visible way, the spinal cord forms with equal numbers of cells along its length but, as many fewer neurones are required to wire up the midriff than are needed to control the muscles of the limbs, the neurones of the spinal cord undergo a wave of cell death, leaving only those cells needed to meet the body's requirements. Even during adult life there are situations in which cell death is required, such as the monthly cycle of cell proliferation followed by cell loss that occurs in the uterus during menstruation.

Cell suicide also protects the body from events that could result in cancer. Many errors in the machinery of the cell that could lead to the beginnings of cancer instead trigger the cell to commit cell suicide for the good of the whole body.

Regardless of the route by which cell suicide is initiated, a programme is activated through which the cell uses its available energy to kill itself in a way that does not disrupt its neighbours. As far as our bodies are concerned, we can live without any given cell; in fact, we can afford to lose very many cells. However, only one cell has to go wrong in a way that leads to cancer and we have a life-threatening disease. It is not surprising that our cells have developed to favour cell death as an emergency exit when they might pass on defective DNA to the next cellular generation. Apoptosis is the last resort for cells: the body's final line of defence against the possibility of cancer. If a cell senses that all is not well, and its continued replication would generate a clone of highly defective cells, it can take the cell suicide option and remove itself from the body.

The ultimate sacrifice

When cell death occurs as part of the normal life of a cell, it is regulated by signals from outside or inside the cells. With respect to cancer, it is mainly the internal triggers of cell death that must be overcome. There are several checkpoints in the cell cycle that determine whether the cell is allowed to complete its replication. Events inside the cell, such as when DNA is so damaged that the cell cannot repair it, are sensed by the gatekeepers, such as P53. If these checkpoints cannot be passed, events can be initiated that irreversibly commit the cell to destroy itself.

The central feature of apoptosis is that it removes the cell from the body without the release of toxic components from within the cell, and so does not cause an inflammatory response. This is achieved by a tightly regulated series of events that destroy the cell from within and activate cells of the immune system to clear up the debris.

The key players in apoptosis are a family of proteins called *caspases*, which can be inhibited by proteins called IAPs, (*i*nhibitors of *a*poptosis). The caspases attack and digest other proteins, causing the degradation of many cellular components. The caspases are both the initiators of cell death and, to a large extent, the cell's executioners. Their role in cell death is often referred to as the *caspase cascade*; once the first caspase is activated, it triggers the activation of the next caspase, and this activates more caspases. This is typical of signalling pathways in the cell; each step in the pathway amplifying the cell's response. A more unusual feature of the caspase cascade is that each caspase activates the next by cutting it in two. In the same way, the final executioner caspases can activate or disrupt other components of the cell by cutting them into several pieces. These final target proteins trigger the hallmark features of this form of cell death, including the breakdown of the DNA into small pieces and the budding-off of small pieces of cell membrane.

At the end of apoptosis, the cell is broken into a series of small, membrane-bound fragments – vesicles – which are engulfed by specialized cells of the immune system. There, they are completely broken down and the components recycled. At no point are the contents of the dying cell released, to be seen by other parts of the immune system. This is why cell death sends out no warning signals to the rest of the body and so no inflammatory response is initiated. The reason such a tidy system evolved is probably because inflammation is both energy-consuming and destructive to nearby tissues.

Evading death

Of all the aspects of a cancer cell's behaviour, cell death is one of the most critical, both to the cancer's formation and to potential therapies. No matter what else has gone wrong in a cell, if that cell were to sense the defect and start its suicide programme, the problem would simply go away. So how do cancer cells evade this form of cell death?

There appear to be two routes by which apoptosis is circumvented in cancer cells. One is through increased levels of anti-apoptotic factors, such as the IAPs. One IAP, survivin, is found in most human tumours, but not in normal cells. The second route is the inactivation of pro-apoptotic factors such as P53. Since P53 is one of the key sensors of DNA damage, which not only inhibits proliferation but can also initiate apoptosis, it is not surprising that P53 mutations are so frequent in cancer. If P53 does not function correctly, the cell in which the DNA is damaged can survive and continue to proliferate. In addition, mutations in many different components of the apoptosis machinery, including the caspases, can also lead to survival of cancer cells when they should normally die.

This particular aspect of a cancer cell's biology is important in several respects. It allows the cancer cells to survive and so allows the cancer to continue to grow. Since one of the mechanisms by which some chemotherapeutic drugs work is the induction of apoptosis, a defect in apoptosis can also make the cancer cells more resistant to those therapies. However, response to therapy does not generally correlate well with the levels of pro- or anti-apoptotic factors, probably because most therapies kill cells in a manner largely independent of apoptosis. Despite this, the cell death machinery is an important target in our attempts to kill cancer cells. If we could overcome the block in the programme that leads to cell death, we could simply trigger cancer cells to remove themselves. This thought has, not surprisingly, occurred to many scientists and is an active avenue of research.

Summary

The cells of a cancer must divide *ad infinitum*. This means that they must avoid entering pathways that stop that division (senescence) or lead to the cells' death (apoptosis). Despite the many genes and proteins that play a part in these processes, the mutation of just a few key genes, such as P53, can be enough to make cells immortal and so achieve a key step in cancer progression.

4
Surviving and spreading

Even after overcoming normal control of the cell cycle and avoiding the signals that tell defective cells to die, such cells would still pose little threat to our health if they remained otherwise normal. They have yet more barriers to overcome simply to survive and, in most cases, cannot kill us unless they can spread to other tissues.

Feeding the tumour

Irrevocably damaged, but doomed to divide and divide, cancer cells produce an ever-growing family of immortal cells. Like any family, they make growing demands for life's essentials: sufficient water, food and oxygen. Tumour cells wouldn't make much impact on our bodies unless they had a supply of these necessities to sustain their growth.

For cells, the bringer of food, water and oxygen is usually the elaborate network of blood vessels that makes up our circulatory system. Without access to this, a rapidly growing tumour would soon run out of resources, starve and suffocate. When a cancer begins to grow, the body's normal network of blood vessels is already fully formed, so the cancer cells must find a way to encourage new blood vessel growth. Unfortunately, as with the control of cell division and cell death, cancers develop ways to overcome this problem and, as a result, quite literally grow *ad nauseam*.

The reason blood vessels develop when and where they do in the normal growing body is that other cells produce substances that either promote or repress their growth. For a cancer to develop to a stage where it becomes a medical problem, it must hijack these mechanisms to ensure that blood vessels begin growing into and around the tumour, providing nourishment for its further growth. This process of blood vessel growth, *angiogenesis*, is essential to the cancer's survival.

Study of this area of cancer biology is relatively new. Thanks largely to the insight of an American doctor and researcher, Judah Folkman, it has become one of the main arms of research into cancer biology. Folkman's insight was to propose, in 1971, that the tumour itself might play a significant role in the process by which it becomes infiltrated by a functional blood supply. It was soon clear that this insight provided a new point of attack for researchers and clinicians to try and starve the tumour to death. Indeed, this is still a major line of development for new therapies (see chapter 13), in which Folkman played a leading role until his death in 2008.

To ensure that they will have a substantial blood supply, cancer cells activate the same systems that the body uses when angiogenesis is necessary under normal conditions. Our blood vessels are lined with a layer of so-called endothelial cells, responsible for the exchange of various molecules between the blood and surrounding tissues and maintaining a robust barrier against leakage. However, given an appropriate stimulus, these cells are able to switch to an alternative state in which they begin to divide and move, generating new branches that grow out from the existing vessels. As with most biological processes, the regulation of these two alternative states is controlled by many different signals, including molecules that promote branching and those that inhibit it. Thus, the cancer has a simple route to ensure that it becomes infiltrated with new blood vessels – it produces those molecules that encourage the sprouting and growth of nearby blood vessels. Many cancers produce such proteins, in particular the protein VEGF. By this means alone, nearby blood vessels are kicked into action.

The stimulated endothelial cells of the blood vessels begin to secrete proteins called *metalloproteinases*. These metalloproteinases are enzymes that eat away the *extracellular matrix*, a mix of proteins and sugars that surrounds our cells. By this means the blood vessels forge a pathway towards and into the tumour mass. The outcome is a very effective extension of the circulatory system, which supplies the tumour with oxygen and nutrients and removes waste products. Without this, the growth of the tumour would be limited to only a few millimetres. By activating growth of the circulatory system, the tumour is able to overcome this restriction on its size and go on to become a more aggressively growing entity, from which it can make its final transition to becoming fully malignant.

The triggering of angiogenesis by molecules such as VEGF does not in general seem to reflect one of the mutational steps required for a cancer to progress. In many tumours, the release of VEGF may simply reflect a normal cellular process designed to ensure that all tissues gain sufficient oxygen. When cells do not have enough oxygen, this activates a series of events that ends with VEGF being switched on. Thus, activation of VEGF is the cell's way of responding to suffocation, by ensuring that the blood supply comes to its rescue. Also, it seems that one of the consequences of activating several of the well-studied oncogenes is that they then cause an increase in VEGF production or decrease inhibition of angiogenesis. Likewise, some tumour suppressors, such as P53, normally promote the expression of angiogenesis inhibitors. Activation of an oncogene or loss of a tumour suppressor can therefore have a dramatic effect on the normal regulation of blood vessel growth, providing the trigger for the tumour cells to encourage those blood vessels to come to their aid.

How cancers spread (metastasis)

In most cases, even a rapidly growing tumour is not a major problem unless the cancer has spread – *metastasized*. A tumour that has not spread can often be removed by surgery and any remaining tumour cells killed by treatments restricted to the tumour site. If a tumour has spread, then chemotherapy is generally needed to reach the cancer cells no matter where they are, and even then some may evade the treatment and so secondary tumours return afterwards. But developing the ability to spread throughout the body is no trivial task for the cell.

The vast majority of deaths from cancer are due to cancers called *carcinomas*. These cancers are derived from epithelial tissues, such as the tissues of the skin or the lining of the gut. Epithelial tissues are tightly associated layers of cells, firmly attached to each other to make a tissue barrier. For such cells to spread to other parts of the body, they must unstick and break out of their normal tissue layer, get into the circulatory system, get back out of the circulatory system, move into a new tissue and then survive and grow in their new location. It is remarkable that any cell ever develops such amazing new powers, but, unfortunately, many cancer cells do. By the end of their days, cancer cells have become hardened criminals, capable of very many acts totally unacceptable to cellular society, including their final escape from the tissue or organ in which they are normally imprisoned. This progress from a benign, confined tumour to an aggressive, invasive cancer can be broken down into four steps.

Step 1: Separation

For a cell to escape from a tumour, it must first unstick itself from its neighbours. Recent evidence suggests that one molecule, E-cadherin, is a key component of the glue that holds cells together. This protein is lost in several classes of cancers. When it is artificially replaced (in an experimental tumour model),

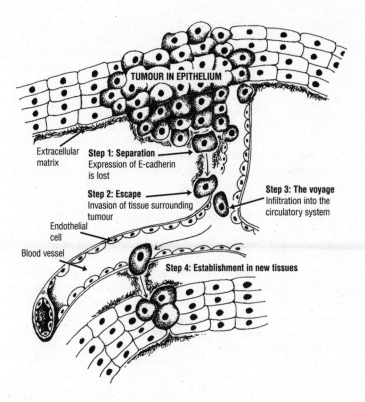

Figure 7 Metastasis of an epithelial tumour

E-cadherin can block the ability of cancer cells to spread. Given the power of this molecule to interfere with the spread of cancer cells, it has become a candidate for therapeutic approaches.

At the core of this behaviour are master control transcription factors that switch a bank of genes on and off, to make the cell change its behaviour. The same master control factors, in particular the *snail* and *slug* proteins, play this role both in normal development and in cancer. It is these proteins that are responsible for switching off E-cadherin in spreading cancer cells.

GENES: THE NAME GAME

Where do gene names come from? Much of our understanding of genes comes from studies of the fruit fly, *Drosophila melanogaster*, and it is in this species that many genes were first named. When the equivalent gene was later discovered in mice, humans or other vertebrates, it was given the same, or a related, name.

Embryonic development is often studied in mutant strains of flies. The name of the gene reflects the way the fly, or its larvae, looked when the function of the gene was disrupted by a mutation. A mutation that caused the fly to develop with an extra segment in its thorax, carrying an extra set of wings, led to the gene being named *bi-thorax*. Mutations in many different genes turned the fly larvae from asymmetric maggots, with one side covered in small hair-like spikes, into symmetrical maggots, either covered entirely in these spikes or entirely without them. Hence, the genes that, when mutated, resulted in larvae covered in these spikes were named *cactus, hedgehog, porcupine, gooseberry* and so on; those genes where mutants completely lacked the spikes were named *tube, torpedo, gurken, pipe* and so on.

What about *snail* and *slug*, the vertebrate genes that control cell adhesion? When the *snail* gene was mutated so that it no longer functioned, the larva's entire internal organs were lost, causing the larva to twist like a snail's shell. Vertebrate versions of this gene were later found and also called *snail*. When a related gene was found, it was called *slug*, to indicate its relationship to the snail gene. In this respect, the name ceases to relate to any function the gene might have.

Another lovely example of this type of naming comes from the *Drosophila* gene, *hedgehog*. When several genes in vertebrates were found to bear a close resemblance to the *Drosophila hedgehog* gene, they were named *desert hedgehog, Indian hedgehog, sonic hedgehog* and *tiggy-winkle hedgehog*. The latter part of the name derives from the *Drosophila* gene from which the family gains its name and the former from the rather weird sense of humour of certain scientists. None of these does anything 'hedgehog-like' in vertebrates!

Step 2: Escape

Even when cells are free to separate from their neighbours, they do not normally move far, trapped by the layers of cells and structures that surround them. Most cells find themselves in a dense and impenetrable environment, the extracellular matrix. To move any distance, cells must not only unstick, but also forge a route through the extracellular matrix. The activation of enzymes, such as the metalloproteinases that can degrade the extracellular matrix, allows cells first to invade the tissue immediately around the tumour and eventually to penetrate into the blood vessels. However, unlike the blood vessels, cancer cells do not themselves produce the enzymes. Instead they hijack metalloproteinases produced by the normal cells of the body. The metalloproteinases are generally produced in an inactive form so the cancer cells are able to subvert them by producing proteins that activate them. The metalloproteinases then digest the extracellular matrix around the tumour, allowing the cancer cells to escape into the body.

Step 3: The voyage

For cancer cells to spread to distant sites in the body and lead to the sort of secondary tumours with which we are all too familiar, they need a means of transport. This is almost always provided by the circulatory system. The infiltration of new blood vessels into the initial tumour therefore turns out to be double trouble. The circulatory system not only provides ready access to nutrients but also an efficient route by which the tumour can spread. The blood vessels that infiltrate tumours are often rather defective and leaky, making it even easier for the cancer cells to enter them.

The circulatory system is not always the main route of escape for tumour cells. Cancer cells sometimes first get into the lymph system, which normally drains fluid from tissues. Although such lymphatic vessels do not infiltrate tumours to the same extent as blood vessels do, they provide an alternative exit route for the tumour cells. The lymph nodes, where cells in the lymph system collect, are frequently one of the first sites where cancer spread is detected. A patient with cancer will often have these nodes checked to determine if the cancer has spread. From the lymph system, the cells could gain access to the blood system and spread throughout the body, and it is via the blood system that most cancer cells appear to spread.

One way or another, the cancer cells reach the blood, but they don't hang about. If small enough, they could make it all the way around the body and back to where they started in about one minute, but most cells do not survive the journey. In an experiment in which cancer cells were labelled and injected into mice, only about one in a thousand cells survived. This sounds like good news, until we realize that a tumour might shed millions of cells into the circulatory system every day. Once cancer cells have acquired the ability to escape from the initial tumour and enter the bloodstream, there is a much greater chance that secondary tumours will occur. But where?

In 1928, James Ewing (co-founder of the American Association for Cancer Research and the Sloan Kettering Cancer Center), already established as one of the foremost cancer researchers in the USA, proposed that the location of secondary tumours was due to mechanical constraints of cell movement. Ewing noted that when cancer cells within the blood reached the next organ through which the circulation passes, they would find themselves entering smaller and smaller blood vessels until they reached the finest vessels, in structures called *capillary beds*. The cancer cells are generally larger than the smallest of these capillaries and so they get stuck. This could explain why secondary tumours often arise at these next stops on the circulatory system. From the stomach and colon, secondary tumours often arise in the next stop, the liver; from breast cancers, the next stop is the lung.

The lung is the last stop before the heart, so cells originating from a primary tumour in the lung can end up almost anywhere (although, in lung cancer, it is the disease in the lung itself that is usually fatal).

Step 4: Pastures new

On arriving at their new location, cancer cells must escape from the blood vessels and enter their new home. This seems to pose little difficulty for the cells: the endothelial cells lining the blood vessels are very co-operative and move aside, allowing the cancer cells to squeeze between them, closing up the gap afterwards. However, not all cancer cells can form a tumour in all the locations in which they come to rest, suggesting there needs to be some kind of recognition between the cancer cells and their new environment before they can become established.

One possible explanation was originally suggested by Stephen Paget in 1889. He attempted to explain the distribution of secondary tumours that had spread from cases of breast cancer. In his still widely accepted 'seed and soil' model, Paget proposed that the initiation of secondary tumours involves a match between the cell that arrives and the environment in which it lands, just as seeds disperse in all directions but only survive in appropriate soil conditions. To his credit, despite the fact that his name is generally linked to this key hypothesis, Paget was keen to point out that others, in particular the Austrian Ernst Fuchs, had already proposed this basic model. We now understand that cells must have specific receptors that allow them to respond to signals in different tissues, thus defining where they are likely to spread. One feature that provides an explanation for the tendency of certain tumours to spread to specific tissues is their adhesion. The very same adhesion systems that glue the cells of the original cancer together might also underlie the ability of those same cells to become established in specific secondary sites, by establishing appropriate interactions with their new neighbours.

In fact, that recognition must go further than simple adhesion. The cells of our body require continuous reassurance to stop them becoming suicidal (chapter 3, p. 34–37). When a cell finds itself in a new environment, like someone suddenly transported to a distant land where they do not speak the language, it does not recognize the signals it receives. Without those reassuring messages, apoptosis might ensue. To survive, a cell must learn the language of its new environment; it must change so that it now responds to its new environment to thrive as a secondary tumour. This change can evolve before the cell emigrates from the original tumour, some cells from the original tumour being better at growing in a new environment than others. Alternatively, tumour cells can improve their ability to survive after they arrive in their new home. This was shown in an experiment in which tumour cells were implanted into a distant tissue location and allowed to grow. Cells from the new tumour were then transplanted into the same tissue in a new animal. Repeating this tumour growth and transplantation several times resulted in the cells becoming much better at establishing tumours than the original cell population. A cancer cell looking for a new location in which to settle down and cause havoc can either get a phrase book in advance or learn the language when it gets there but to get by in the first few days, it must arrive with a basic ability to communicate.

Who was right? Do cancer cells form secondary tumours when they get trapped in the capillaries, as Ewing suggested, or do they form tumours only where they find an environment in which they can thrive, as proposed by Paget? It seems that both explanations are true; most secondary tumours develop in the next location where the cells get stuck in the tiny blood vessels of the capillary beds, as long as those cells can thrive in that environment. The probability of secondary tumours arising in a given tissue is a balance between the likelihood of cells becoming trapped there and the level of match between the seed (cancer cell) and soil (new tissue). Given the importance of the match between the cancer cell and its new environment, Paget's final statement, in his paper of 1889, remains as apt as it ever has been. In addition to the study of the cancer cells themselves (the seed), he wrote, 'observations of the properties of the soil may also be useful'.

Defence

One aspect of the tissue environment that we might hope would protect us from rogue cancer cells is the body's immune system. This is especially true when the cancer cells enter the blood, where the front line troops of this defence lie in wait. Why then are cancer cells not eradicated by this, our main line of defence against most diseases?

The immune system is designed to recognize and destroy alien entities that have invaded our bodies. It is specifically designed *not* to attack our own cells and, of course, cancers are made up of our own cells. Our immune systems depend upon this ability to recognize 'self' from 'non-self'. If this does not happen properly and our immune cells see some of our own cells or proteins as non-self, these targets are attacked and autoimmune disease may develop, as happens in diseases such as coeliac disease, diabetes mellitus type 1 or rheumatoid arthritis. For this reason, cancers are, especially in their early stages, relatively invisible to the immune system.

It is true that the immune system does generally fail us with respect to cancer, but it is far from useless; without it, we might develop cancer much more often. Evidence for this comes from experiments in which the immune system was disrupted experimentally in mice. This led to a significant increase in the incidence of cancer development. Similar observations have been made in humans: when people have a kidney or liver transplant they are treated with agents to suppress their immune system, to reduce the chances of their body rejecting the transplanted organ. It seems that one side effect of these treatments is an increase in the occurrence of certain cancers (as much as two or three times that of the general population). This effect may not be entirely due to reduced immune targeting of tumour cells. The cancers that arise are also more commonly those caused by a viral infection than normally expected, so a reduced immune response to the viruses probably plays some part. However, reduced targeting of tumour cells by the immune system is certainly a major issue, since the outcome for transplant patients who do develop cancer (or have a history of cancer) tends to be much worse than would normally be expected. Of course, the benefits of these treatments far outweigh any increase in the risk of cancer.

It seems that many, probably most, cells that escape the primary tumour and enter the bloodstream are hunted down and destroyed by cells of the immune system known as natural killer cells. This protection by our immune systems is called *immunosurveillance*. The reason the immune system can identify and kill many cancer cells, especially in these later stages of cancer, is because while cancer cells are indeed our own cells, they are not normal. Because cancer cells become abnormal, they acquire proteins, *tumour associated antigens*, on their surfaces that the immune system may never have seen before and so the immune cells will attack them. These tumour associated antigens might be the products of mutated genes or may just be inappropriately or over-expressed proteins.

Unfortunately, while this does allow many tumour cells to be destroyed, this immune response is not normally strong enough to cause the tumour's complete destruction. There are several reasons for this. One is the simple fact that the proteins on the surface of tumour cells are not so different from normal cells. In addition, cancer cells can change under the 'selective pressure' of the immune system. This is very like the laws of evolution – any cell that develops in a way that makes it less recognizable to the immune system (so called *immunoediting*) will have a 'selective advantage' and so it might outgrow the other cells of the tumour. However, it also seems that tumours often release signalling proteins, such as VEGF, that can actually subdue the immune response. Many of the most recent developments in cancer therapy are aimed at combatting this ability of the cancer cells to escape the attention of the immune system. The nature of these inhibitory molecules and the approaches being developed to combat them are discussed in chapter 13, p. 160–161.

So while our immune system does its best to fight off the cancer cells, especially when they spread through our blood, the cancer cells normally win the battle.

Summary

Many potentially cancerous growths never become fully malignant. A large number of benign growths remain small and stop growing because they are limited by a lack of nutrients and oxygen. In order to overcome this limitation new blood vessels must grow into the tumour to carry these essential supplies to its cells. For those tumours that do develop a blood supply, the final and most pernicious stage of their development, generally quite a late step, is to develop the ability to spread beyond the tissue in which they first appeared. For most types of cancer, it is the spread of the cancer that is finally fatal.

Part 2
The enemy forces

5

Mutation, mutation, mutation

For a cell to become so abnormal as to be described as a cancer, it must undergo many changes. A benign tumour can proliferate when it should not and avoid dying when it should, but only when the cells of the tumour acquire the additional ability to induce the growth of new blood vessels and make the many changes needed to spread do they qualify as cancer cells.

How can so many of the complex processes that normally control the cell be disrupted in cancer? What exactly goes wrong? In one respect, all these errors in cell behaviour are the same: our genes are to blame.

Although each of our cells has only two copies of each gene, they have many copies of the proteins. When a cell divides, the genes are replicated, so that two copies of each gene can be passed on to each new daughter cell. If a mistake exists in one copy of any gene, it is copied and inherited by one of the two daughter cells. Only DNA is inherited in this way, and so only mistakes in the DNA are passed on from one cellular generation to the next. While damage to the DNA code will cause the defect to be inherited by later generations, damage to the proteins is not passed on. When cells divide, the proteins they contain are inherited by the daughter cells, but these will gradually decay and be replaced in each generation of cells by new proteins based on the sequences of the genes that the cells have inherited.

The events that initiate the path of a cell towards eventual cancer begin when one of a small number of key genes (such as those that control proliferation or cell death – see chapters 2 and 3) is damaged and not repaired, and that damaged gene is inherited by the progeny of that cell. Fortunately, mutations in such key genes are very rare, but on the occasions when they do occur the march towards a possible cancer has begun. However, full-blown cancer only arises when several processes are disrupted in a single cell, so mutations in several genes are needed.

How successive mutations cause a cell to progress from normal cell, through benign stages of excess proliferation, to fully malignant cancer is very much like the process of evolution as described by Charles Darwin, resulting from a series of random changes to genes combined with survival of the fittest cell. The first mutation usually leads to one cell dividing more quickly than its neighbours; this produces a clone of daughter cells that begin to form a growing mass. Further random mutations within that growing clone of cells may result in one of them becoming even more abnormal, perhaps dividing even more quickly or becoming better able to survive, while its neighbours might slow down or die. And so it goes on, each successive mutation making one cell even stronger at each step, giving it a competitive advantage over its neighbours. The final aggressive cancer cells are the descendants of a lineage of cells that has benefited from the most advantageous series of changes.

These mutational events are very rare; the reason several mutations occur in a single cell is because one of the first mutations increases the chances of subsequent mutations. This is because the processes that are disrupted by mutations in cancer-causing genes include the machinery that protects those cells from acquiring more mutations. As more mutations are acquired, this makes further mutations even more likely. Thus, as the cancer progresses, its DNA and genes become ever more damaged. The result is a cell with a very unstable genome, often incurring multiple breaks and reorganisation of the chromosomes. Such massive damage to the genome is almost invariably evident by

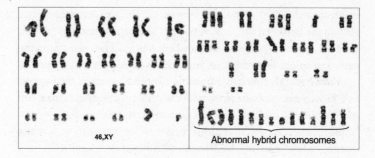

Figure 8 The abnormal genome of cancers
On the left is a 'spread' of the normal chromosomes of one human cell showing the two copies of each chromosome, one originally derived from that person's mother and the other from their father. On the right is a chromosomal spread from a cancer cell showing multiple irregularities including new 'hybrid' chromosomes, resulting from chromosome breakage and inaccurate repair, composed of parts from two or more different chromosomes. In addition, this cell is so abnormal that it has more than the normal two copies of some chromosomes.

the time a malignant cancer is diagnosed. Analysis of the chromosomes within the cells of such cancers reveals horrendous distortion of their form, with some fragments missing and other fragments added, broken or reattached in the wrong place, like a child's attempt to fix a vase they have accidentally smashed. The result is the disruption of many genes and, as a consequence, many aspects of cell behaviour, revealed in the malignant cancer's aggressive growth.

What are the odds?

It is painfully clear that cancer is not a rare disease. Post-mortem studies show that, by the age of 85, about 85% of men have developed prostate cancer. In women, although no similar analysis has been carried out, the dramatic increase in the incidence of almost all cancers between the ages of 65 and 85 suggests that, given long enough, almost all of us would develop cancer. The odds of getting cancer are therefore about once per human body per 100 years.

However, due to the number of events that must occur for a cell to achieve such an abnormal state, the individual cancer cell itself is indeed rare. A cancer cell does not arise every one in a million cells, nor even one in every million million. It actually occurs in fewer than 1 in 10 million million (ten trillion – 10^{13}) cells, which is the approximate number of cells in our bodies. If each cell were a person, this would be the equivalent of one person going wrong in the population of one thousand earths. In other words, it is very, very rare for a cell to go so wrong that it can form a malignant cancer. Unfortunately, we have so very many cells in our bodies that even such a rare event is enough to lead to, on average, one cancer in each of us if we lived to 100.

It is actually not unusual for cells to make some of the mistakes that might contribute to becoming cancerous, but most of these fail to progress to a full-blown cancer. We all contain small pockets of cells that can grow in a benign way, but will typically do no more than that during our lifetimes. The most evident are our moles and skin tags (as discussed in Chapter 3 p. 33, chapter 7 p.79). Many of us will also develop polyps, small growths on the surface of our gut. Although on rare occasions these do progress to full-blown colon cancer, in most cases they do not. The longer we live, the more time there is for cells to be affected in this way, and the more we notice the appearance of such blemishes. Clearly, then, the initiation of tumour growth is not so rare, but in any given cell progression to more aggressive stages is very unlikely, because the chance of additional critical mutations arising in a cell that has already incurred one mutation is still rare. Even if a cell does acquire more mutations, relatively few genes play roles so central to regulating cell behaviour that their mutation can contribute to cancerous growth. Despite the large number of these benign growths from which we all suffer, only about one in three of us will get cancer (although recent estimates suggest that this could be nearer to one in two of those born after 1960). This is either through bad luck or through failing to avoid the risks that encourage those cells to acquire further mutations. The rest of us will instead die of something else before the, otherwise inevitable, cancer occurs.

What causes the mutations that lead to cancer? To a large extent, we all know the answer. Even if you only reply 'smoking', you have already answered this question for as many as 40,000 cancer deaths per year in Britain, over 160,000 in the USA and about 1,000,000 per year worldwide. As many as one in three of all male cancer deaths in developed countries is a direct result of smoking tobacco. We could substantially reduce the number of cancer deaths simply by eradicating the use of tobacco. This seems unlikely to happen and, even if it did, we are still left with a very large number of cancers. That is why we need to understand how various carcinogenic agents can result in the features we associate with cancer.

Cancer results from damage to our genes. Of all the observations from decades of intensive research into cancer, this is the most central and definitive. To understand why we get cancer, we need to understand how our DNA, the chemical from which our genes are made, can be damaged.

The way we live exposes us to many attacking forces, from the sun's ultraviolet light, to aspects of our diet, to more avoidable agents, such as cigarette smoke. These agents cause mutations to arise in our genomes, not by targeting genes that cause cancer but by increasing the random occurrence of mutations throughout our DNA. This increases the probability of a mutation affecting a key gene that can then cause the progress towards cancer to begin. Whatever the cause, DNA damage has the potential to initiate and then advance the progress of a cell towards a cancer.

However, the legions of adversaries laying siege to our precious genomes are matched by an equally impressive battery of defensive artillery and engineering teams, primed to repel and neutralize

Table 1 The causes of cancer

Carcinogen	Types of cancer	Number of cancers worldwide per year	Estimated number of cancer deaths world-wide per year
Tobacco smoke	Lung, mouth, larynx (voice box), oesophagus (food pipe), liver, pancreas, stomach, kidney, bladder and cervix, some types of leukaemia	Lung 1.2 million	1 million (up to 5–6 million from all smoking-related disease)
Cooked foods/ obesity/alcohol	Colon, stomach, mouth, oesophagus and breast		1.5–3 million
Micro-organisms	Stomach, liver and cervical cancer	2 million	1.5 million
Radon	Lung cancer	110,000	100,000
Ultraviolet radiation	melanoma	160,000	50,000
Asbestos	Mesothelioma*	6,000	6,000

Note: These are broad estimates of the numbers and types of cancer caused by some of the most common carcinogens. Together, these may account for over 60% of cancer-related deaths. These numbers are a consensus from the cancer research and healthcare community. Estimates vary widely, so the values should neither be considered accurate nor necessarily accepted by everyone, but are generally conservative estimates. However, the general magnitude and rank order is likely to be correct. The value for the contribution of diet to cancer is a very rough estimate, since the association is much harder to study than for other, simpler, agents.

* No statistics on mesothelioma are available for most countries, so its figure is likely to be a gross underestimate. In the USA and Europe, there are 20 to 30 cases of mesothelioma per 1,000,000 people, suggesting the real numbers worldwide could be over 50,000.

attacking forces and locate and repair any damage they inflict before it can cause long-term ill effects. There are independent sets of repair machinery for each type of DNA damage and sometimes several for one type (this complicated process is described in more detail in Appendix 2). Fortunately, for most of us, our cells are very good at repairing damage to our DNA and the complicated machinery normally runs like clockwork (described in more detail in Appendix 2). When it does not, we are in serious trouble.

How our DNA gets damaged

To understand why we get cancer, the key areas to consider are how our DNA is damaged and why that damage sometimes results in the formation and inheritance of mutations during cell division.

Substantial DNA damage is a hallmark of almost all cancer cells. DNA damage is the mechanism that causes cancer to start and the driving force that makes it progressively worse. Replication of the cell's DNA is an essential step in acquiring DNA mutations. In a normal, healthy, dividing cell, the entire DNA genome is replicated in just a few hours. This is all the more remarkable when one considers that this process requires many proteins, including enzymes that unwind the DNA and others that break and then repair the DNA strands (to avoid them becoming tangled) as well as many accessory proteins needed to load the replication machinery on to the DNA properly and ensure its efficient progress (Appendix 1, p. 181–182).

Despite this remarkable and complex activity, mistakes are rare, because an even larger number of cellular proteins are dedicated to checking and repairing DNA during replication. In the absence of carcinogens, mistakes in the copying process escape the surveillance of the repair machinery only once in every ten million bases. Because of the number of specific events that need to occur in a single cell for cancer to develop, this rate of error is not usually enough to cause cancer. For cancer to occur, something must increase the number of errors: that something is the action of carcinogens. Carcinogens increase the number of damaging events that need to be repaired and some of the resulting mutations can also disrupt the repair processes themselves so that even more mutations are inherited by the next generation of cells.

Despite the potentially disastrous effects of errors in our DNA sequence, most mutations do not cause a problem. This is because, although we each have about 20–25,000 genes (it is surprisingly hard to be sure precisely how many genes there are), these represent less than 3% of our genome. Therefore, about 97% of mutations are likely to be outside those genes, most hitting DNA that has no known function. Although about 20% of the genome seems to have no real function, we really don't know what all the other DNA does, so it is also likely that some mutations will affect other functions of the genome that we don't understand and so contribute to cancer in this way. In addition, only a small proportion of mutations within genes actually disrupt their function, because most changes to a gene do not change the structure of the protein it codes for. Finally, changes in the activity of the vast majority of our 20,000 or so genes do not affect processes that could promote cancer.

It would be very rare indeed for a mutation to play a role in cancer formation. However, if mutations occur frequently enough, some will disrupt genes that could play a role in the progress towards cancer. In general, there are two types of effect. Firstly, a change in the base sequence of the DNA strands could change the structure of the protein for which the gene encodes, which could in turn affect its function, either increasing or decreasing its activity. Alternatively, the altered DNA could affect the control of a gene, either increasing or decreasing the amount of that protein that is made and, at its most extreme, locking the gene into an always on or always off position. If such changes affect a gene that is important in promoting or repressing behaviours that are typical of a cancer cell (such as proliferation, cell death or DNA repair) this mutation will be one step towards cancer.

DNA repair: good intentions, disastrous outcomes

In cancer, it seems that events really do conspire against us. The two competing forces of increased DNA-damaging events and the machinery that is trying to repair it both act against us. The errors that occur during the process of repair create the mutations that are inherited when the cell divides. This tendency of our cells to fight to survive damage is, in some senses, the real cause of cancer. If a very large proportion of our cells were to die due to DNA breaks, this would be a problem to our bodies but we could never-the-less lose a substantial number of cells without it causing any major problems. It is the rather unnecessary, but valiant, attempts of our cells to keep going, even under the onslaught of major genome damage, that generate mutations and so lead to cancer.

An almost universal event during the development of cancer is that one mutation will be within one of the genes that normally ensures that DNA repair is successfully completed. This results in a less effective repair process and so, as further rounds of cell division take place, more DNA damage evades repair and so more mutations arise in other genes needed for DNA repair. In this way the cells enter a downward spiral that all started with one unfortunate random hit in a gene that was supposed to be there to protect us.

Carcinogenesis: the causes of cancer

Our environment plays a major role in our chances of developing cancer. Because exposure to different carcinogens varies in different parts of the world, the types of cancer we are likely to develop depends very much on where we live. If we live in America or the UK, we are much more likely to develop cancer of the colon than the stomach, whereas in Japan stomach cancer is more common. A strong indication that this geographical variation in the incidence of cancer is due to our environment, not our ethnic origins, is that the first generation of children born to Japanese families who settled in the USA switch to the cancer susceptibility typical of their new home. Similarly, liver cancer is widespread in Asian people, but this risk is dramatically reduced in people of Asian descent who are born in the USA.

The agents that cause cancer can be divided into three classes: chemical carcinogens, radiation and infectious agents. In Western countries, chemicals and radiation have the greatest impact; both act by damaging our DNA. However, viruses play a much greater role in some regions, especially the Far East and some less developed countries (see chapter 8).

Summary

It is DNA mutations that cause cancer because they disrupt cell biology and they are inherited from cell generation to cell generation. As cancers progress, more and more mutations are acquired, and so the behaviour of the cells becomes more and more abnormal. Although some errors are made during all DNA replication, it is only the dramatically increased rate of these errors caused by carcinogens that can explain the vast number of cancers that we see in the human population. Only when cells try to divide, replicating their DNA, does the damage caused by carcinogens sometimes result in a change to the sequence of the DNA. These changes are the mutations that have the potential to affect genes and so cause cancer.

6

Chemical carcinogens

Chemical carcinogens are the major cause of cancer that most of us will experience. They can be divided into two classes: those that are very well established, bad in every sense and to be avoided, such as tobacco smoke and asbestos, and those that are an almost inevitable part of everyday life, such as most food-related carcinogens.

Many chemicals can cause cancer, but there are relatively few that we are foolish, or unfortunate, enough to come into contact with at dangerous levels. By far the most important source of chemical carcinogens, in human health terms, is tobacco smoke, although others – exemplified by asbestos – are significant, either because people were exposed to them before we understood their ill effects or because we have failed to eradicate them, for social or economic reasons.

One way that chemicals in our environment can lead to mutations is to cause a chemical change in one of the four types of bases (A, G, C and T) in our DNA (chapter 2, p. 19–20). In a non-dividing cell, these changes will have little effect, because such small changes leave most of the information in the genome available and allow the cell to continue to function. However, in a dividing cell, that DNA must be copied. When the copying machinery reaches the altered region, it cannot read and replicate the DNA sequence correctly. Although the DNA repair machinery is usually able to correct the fault, the more faults there are, the more the mistakes that escape repair and an error in the DNA sequence is introduced. The result is one or more bases being replaced by a wrong base in the next generation of cells and this mutation then being inherited by all future cells produced from that cell. These chemical modifications of individual bases can also have a more dramatic effect, resulting in the DNA replication machinery skipping a base and deleting it in subsequent cellular generations. Among the chemicals that cause such DNA damage, none has had more impact than tobacco smoke.

Tobacco and the causes of lung cancer

Of all cancers, lung cancer is one of the most avoidable. The cause of most cases is clear: smoking tobacco. Tobacco smoke contains about 60 chemicals considered to be carcinogens, most notably the *polycyclic hydrocarbons*. These chemicals are *alkylating agents* that cause the formation of DNA adducts (chemical alterations to the DNA, such as the addition of a methyl [CH_3] group) and therefore cause DNA mutations.

According to Cancer Research UK, smoking tobacco is the UK's 'single greatest cause of preventable illness and early death'. About one in three of the deaths caused by smoking tobacco is due to cancer, of which most are lung cancers. Smoking is also the main preventable cause of cancer of the bladder, mouth and oesophagus (food pipe), and plays a major role in many cases of cancer of the stomach, pancreas, kidney, larynx (voice box), liver, cervix and some types of leukaemia. Most other smoking-related deaths result from heart disease and emphysema (a chronic obstructive lung disease).

Tobacco smoking is responsible for up to 30% of cancer-related deaths in developed countries. The increase in incidence of lung cancer from the 1940s reflects the increase in smoking that started at the beginning of the twentieth century, just after the cigarette-rolling machine was invented in 1881. The 15- to 30-year time lag reflects the time required for the initial carcinogenic event to result in a clinically diagnosed cancer. After a peak in the 1950s, the number of people smoking in the USA, UK and several other economically developed countries began to decline, with a dramatic fall noted since the early 1970s. The effect of this has been a decline in lung cancer rates 20 to 30 years later: since the 1970s, the incidence of lung cancer has begun to drop in these countries and (thanks also to improvements in diagnosis and treatment) lung cancer-related deaths are likewise dropping dramatically. By 2005, the proportion of men dying from lung cancer in the UK was back to the level seen in 1950 and numbers have continued to drop since then to well under half the peak rate seen in the 1970s.

This should be positive news, but sadly these statistics relate only to men and only in some developed countries. Women took up smoking later in the twentieth century, so that, in the West, lung cancer incidence in women began to increase significantly in the 1960s (following a dramatic increase in smoking during the 1940s). The incidence of lung cancer in women continues to rise. Lung cancer is now the most common cause of cancer-related deaths in women in some countries in the West (although breast cancer remains the biggest cause of cancer-related deaths for women worldwide). If current trends continue, by about 2020 more women than men will develop the disease.

Another worrying aspect of recent trends is that, in many countries, the young are now smoking more than the old, the legacy of which we can expect to see as they reach middle age. It is already clear that, although lung cancer is amongst the most rapidly declining class of cancers in men, the incidence is still slowly increasing in women over 60 years of age in the UK. Although rates of lung cancer in younger women are not increasing, in many countries the number of teenage girls and young women who smoke is on the rise and is now similar to the number of young male smokers, so the rate of lung cancer in women is also likely to continue rising in relation to men for the foreseeable future.

Worldwide, the situation is even less promising. The overall number of smokers is increasing rapidly in the Far East and many developing countries, so lung cancer rates also continue to rise steadily. It has been estimated that one-third of the young male population of China will die as a result of tobacco use. This continuing epidemic of smoking has led to predictions that between 10 million and 100 million people will die of tobacco-related disease over the next 30 years, mostly in less-developed countries. This outnumbers the deaths from AIDS, tuberculosis, car accidents, homicide and suicide combined.

Simply not smoking would currently avoid about 150,000 cancer-related deaths per year in the USA alone and about 1,000,000 cancer deaths worldwide. However, given current estimates of 1.3 billion smokers in the world and a time lag of 15 to 30 years for the benefits of reduced smoking levels to be seen, lung cancer is likely to remain a problem for many years to come.

The rise in popularity of alternatives to traditional cigarettes, such as e-cigarettes, provides hope that the number of people smoking tobacco might fall more rapidly. A 2015 study in the UK found that as many as 15% of smokers already use e-cigarettes, and about half of them do so in order to quit smoking tobacco. However, the effects of such alternatives on our health are still not fully tested. Although almost certainly less toxic than smoking tobacco, they are still likely to carry some risks.

Another recently identified problem is that many cases of lung cancer in women in the Far East do not appear to be attributable to tobacco smoke at all. In Southeast Asia as many as half the women who develop lung cancer have never smoked. Analysis of the genomes of the cancers in these women shows that the damage to their genes does not look like the sort that is caused by the carcinogens in tobacco. In these cases, the evidence suggests that the most likely culprit is exposure to carcinogens that are released when cooking food at high temperatures in oil in poorly ventilated spaces, although general air pollution may also contribute to these cases.

Asbestos

Asbestos was first widely used at the end of the nineteenth century. Its fire-retardant properties and fibrous nature, which allow it to be woven, made it an ideal material for applications as diverse as oven gloves and roof insulation. Unfortunately, asbestos also readily releases a powder of microscopic fibres that can be inhaled.

The most immediate consequence of exposure to asbestos is *asbestosis*, a disease in which these fibres cause scarring of the lung, and by the 1940s it was well established that workers in the asbestos industry also suffered increased rates of lung cancer (by the early 21st century asbestos exposure appears to account for more than 1 in 20 cases of lung cancer).

By the late 1950s, it became apparent that asbestos also caused an otherwise rare cancer, *mesothelioma*, a cancer of the linings of the lungs, chest and abdomen. Mesothelioma is linked to those who have suffered significant exposure to asbestos and this remains its only known cause.

The mechanism by which asbestos fibres cause mesothelioma is unusual. The tiny fibres penetrate the cells of the lung and gut and pass through into the body cavities surrounding them. There, they cause an inflammatory response, believed to be the cause of the cancer formation. In fact, inflammation may play a significant role in many cancers, although the reasons why are not entirely clear. However, it is clear that part of the inflammatory response is to inhibit cell death and promote cellular proliferation, both key aspects of tumour cell behaviour.

Although our understanding of the risks of asbestos has now led to established policies for avoiding its use in developed countries, it remains the cause of an increasing number of cancer deaths, due to exposure before this awareness developed. Even now, approximately 10–15,000 asbestos-related cancer deaths are reported each year in the USA and as many as 5,000 in the UK. The subsequent increase in the incidence of mesothelioma, despite a dramatic decrease in asbestos exposure, stands as evidence of the slow progress of this illness, from the time one is exposed to a carcinogen and the time when cancer is first detected. However, since 2005, rates have begun to decrease in the UK and Europe. The rates in the US have also been declining since the late 1990s.

Unlike smoking, there is no pleasure to be gained from asbestos. Neither can it be considered addictive, so we might think it is a cause of cancer that we can readily avoid. Unfortunately, there is much money to be made from mining and trading asbestos, and this gives some people a great deal of pleasure. Asbestos production, largely by companies based in Russia, Kazakhstan, China, India and Brazil, continues unabated at the time of writing (the last mines in Canada ceased production in 2011, although the Canadian government still refuse to join those that want to classify asbestos as a dangerous substance). The use of asbestos has been banned in many developed countries, so its sale and use are now concentrated in countries where it is produced and in some less-developed nations. It seems cynical, at the very least, for such a trade to continue when the consequences of asbestos use have led to its removal from buildings and an end to its use in the building trade in the West. Indeed, its use is banned in the European Union, Japan, Australia and several other countries, although many have yet to join them. As recently as November

2015, doctors and health experts in Canada asked their president to ban the use of asbestos.

The price of a good meal

Does what we eat affect our chances of getting cancer? Yes: it can both increase and decrease our probability of developing cancer. So, it appears to be true that if we eat all the right things and none of the wrong things our chances of developing cancer will be significantly reduced.

The monks who live in the monasteries of Mount Athos in Greece lead long and exceptionally healthy lives. This is believed to reflect their unusual lifestyle, in particular their diet. The monks eat no red meat and only occasionally fish; they live primarily on home-grown vegetables, fruit and pulses, together with rice, pasta and bread. On many days they eat only one, vegan, meal. Although this is anecdotal and far from being a controlled scientific study, they have been reported to suffer almost no lung, bowel or bladder cancer and have exceptionally low levels of heart disease and other diseases of ageing. Also, despite living into very old age (up to 104 years), reports suggest that they show very low rates of prostate cancer, a disease that otherwise seems almost inevitable for most men.

It has been estimated that our diet is responsible for about one-third of cancers, although identifying the good and bad parts of our diet is not a precise science. It is very difficult to be certain that a given food is a definite culprit, since it may be just one part of a particular lifestyle.

So, what are the carcinogens that we eat? Few of the chemicals we ingest are actual carcinogens. Most are seen by the body simply as toxins; chemicals that are poisonous to the body that should be got rid of as rapidly as possible. Many toxins must be modified to make them soluble and thus more easily excreted;

this is where things go wrong. CYPs (cytochrome P450 enzymes), found in the liver, trigger the modification of such toxins. Unfortunately, the actions of some CYPs, which should save us from the nasty cellular toxicity of these chemicals, back-fire on the cellular community as a whole. Many of these toxins generally have no ill effect on our genomes until CYPs convert them to a more reactive form, creating carcinogens that attack our DNA.

Despite the difficulty in identifying specific problem foods, there is good evidence that processed red meat is a source of carcinogens. The aptly named EPIC (European Prospective Investigation into Cancer) study analysed the diets of over 500,000 Europeans, including 1,300 people who suffered from bowel cancer. In 2005, the researchers reported that the one significant risk factor shown by the study was the eating of large amounts of red meat, which was implicated in stomach and colon cancer. In October 2015, a report from the World Health Organization presented their analysis of all available studies on the relationship between diet and cancer. They found that diets high in processed red meat could be responsible for as many as 50,000 cancer deaths per year worldwide (that's about 20 times less than tobacco). They estimated that every 50 grams of processed meat eaten daily increased the risk of colon cancer by 18%, i.e. if you eat an average of 100gm of processed meat every day your risk of developing colon cancer in the UK increases from about 7–10%. Looked at this another way, it has been esti-mated that about one in five cases of colon cancer are due to eating red and processed meats. Although we cannot be certain what it is about red meat that underlies this carcinogenic activity, cooking, especially at high temperatures (such as frying or barbe-cuing), is known to convert chemicals in the meat into *hetero-cyclic amines*. These chemicals are not carcinogenic in their own right, but become so when activated by the CYPs in the liver. These activated compounds are sufficiently stable to survive long enough to leave the liver and move to other organs where cancer could then arise. On a brighter note, the EPIC study identified fibre, folate, calcium, vitamin B and vitamin D as dietary factors that reduced the risk of colon or rectal cancer.

Until the last decade, alcohol was not generally regarded as one of the most potent carcinogens but it has now been implicated in the development of several types of cancer. Its greatest impact is seen in cancers of the digestive tract, especially the oesophagus, but it also seems to contribute to the occurrence of cancers of the liver and breast. It has been estimated that alcohol is responsible for as many as 4% of all cancers, including almost 5,000 cases of bowel cancer. For some, alcohol poses a particular threat. Some people – as many as one in three people living in Japan, Taiwan or Korea – have a defective version of the enzyme *alcohol dehydrogenase 2*, one of the enzymes that break down alcohol. Normally, alcohol is broken down in several stages, ending up as harmless substances like carbon dioxide and water. In people with the defective gene, the breakdown of alcohol stops after it is converted to acetaldehyde, which is a carcinogen. This build-up of acetaldehyde is also the cause of *alcohol flushing*, in which the person's face reddens rapidly after they have drunk alcohol. If these people drink large amounts of alcohol they can be as much as 10 times more likely to develop cancers of the mouth and digestive tract. It has been calculated that if all those who exhibit alcohol flushing – and therefore carry the defective gene – were to become light drinkers, as many as 50% of oesophageal cancers in the Japanese male population would be avoided.

Two dietary components that have attracted attention as 'anti-cancer' agents are curcumin (a component of the spice turmeric, well established as a traditional medicine for a wide range of disorders) and green tea. Both may protect us from cancer as well as providing potential therapies for those already diagnosed. Certain cancers, such as colon, breast and prostate, have been observed to be less prevalent in countries where high levels of curcumin are consumed and it has been shown to prevent certain types of cancer in animal models (the mechanisms are not yet entirely clear). Curcumin has now been used in Phase I clinical trials (tested on a small number of people) and has proved to be of low toxicity. However, it appears that curcumin can only reach a sufficient concentration to kill cancer cells while it is actually in the gut, since it is rapidly broken down and therefore does not reach other organs. This means it may have particular benefit in the prevention or even treatment of cancers of the digestive tract, but trials are as yet inconclusive.

Although the case for teas is far from proven, it is clear that the *polyphenols* they contain can inhibit tumour formation and growth in animal models and there is some evidence they could play a similar role in humans. It also seems these chemicals are more readily released from green tea than from black tea. Much larger human studies will be needed to determine if such a common dietary component can help in the fight against cancer.

It seems that good chemicals outweigh the bad ones in some foods but in others the reverse is true. With respect to cancer, bad chemicals come in quite a range of forms, generally involving highly reactive molecules, such as *free radicals* (explained in detail in chapter 7, p. 83). Anything that might react with DNA and change its form is likely to be able to act as a carcinogen. The good chemicals are often those that in some way mop up the reactive molecules and neutralize them. Given that we are certain to ingest some level of toxins along with the good stuff, even in good foods, what are our cells doing about it?

They are not unprepared. The first line of defence against ingested carcinogens is made up of chemicals that react with any highly reactive molecules, rendering them harmless. These include vitamins C and E, although the benefits of taking vitamin C supplements have always been controversial; recent studies have raised concerns that it may have some detrimental effects on standard therapies. Our cells also possess enzymes specifically designed to inactivate free radicals. One such enzyme is superoxide dismutase, which converts highly reactive *superoxide* molecules into the comparatively harmless hydrogen peroxide. Another major line of defence is the glutathione S-transferases (GSTs), which chemically link potential carcinogens to another chemical, glutathione. This makes them unreactive and they can be further degraded and excreted. The importance of this system explains why inactivation of the genes encoding GSTs is seen in several types of cancer, suggesting that the inactivation of this type of enzyme strongly predisposes for the initiation and progress of these cancers by making the cells more prone to the effects of carcinogens.

The growing problem of obesity also has an impact on cancer; it has been associated with increases in the risk of developing many different cancers, including cancers of the oesophagus, breast, uterus, bowel, pancreas and kidney. These include some of the most common and most deadly of cancers. It has been estimated that in the UK as many as 1 in 20 cancers may be associated with being overweight. However, being obese increases our chances of dying from diseases such as heart attack far more than it does cancer, so, perversely, it may actually reduce our risk of dying from cancer – we may not live long enough for cancer to kill us.

We would all like to know what are 'good' and 'bad' foodstuffs so that we could eat the ideal diet to avoid cancer. Unfortunately, we do not have a clear view of what is good and bad, largely due to the difficulty of untangling our very mixed food intake. Although we are beginning to identify some of the key carcinogens, it is clear that our diet is so complex that many are unlikely ever to become apparent. It seems likely, however, that eating lots of fruit and vegetables and avoiding processed red meats (especially when overcooked) would go some way to reducing our chances of developing several types of cancers.

Summary

Chemical carcinogens are the most prevalent cause of cancer. They come from a wide range of sources and their effects depend upon the tissues to which they have access. Some are relatively mild while others are much more powerful either due to the highly reactive nature of the chemicals themselves or their level of access to cells and their DNA. Tobacco smoke is amongst the worst of these in terms of the large number of highly reactive chemicals it contains and its level of impact directly on the cells of the lungs. Despite the fact that we now know many of the chemicals that we should avoid, progress in reducing the number of cancers in the population are limited by resistance to messages to avoid carcinogens and by the 15 years or more that it takes for the benefits to be seen.

7

Radiation

Other than chemical carcinogens, radiation is the most prevalent cause of cancer. This comes in several forms, ranging from the relatively low-energy ultraviolet light from the sun to the very high-energy radiation from radioactive materials. These are forms of *ionising radiation*, which means that they have sufficient energy to cause electrons to detach from atoms or molecules. Some forms of radiation, such as sunlight, are almost unavoidable, whereas most of us are unlikely to encounter significant levels of most others. Despite this, many people develop cancer as a direct result of exposure to radiation.

Sunlight

When most of us think about radiation, we probably think of nuclear bombs or nuclear waste, but, since we rarely come into contact with these, they contribute very little to the cases of cancer we are likely to encounter. The most prevalent cancer-causing radiation is sunlight: almost all skin cancers appear to be caused by ultraviolet light. If cells are subject to enough ultraviolet light, the energy from this radiation can cause a chemical reaction within the DNA, causing adjacent C and T bases to become chemically linked to form *pyrimidine dimers*. Because of the shape of these abnormal dimers, the DNA replication machinery can misread them. In the most common dimer, C-C, one or both Cs will be converted to a T. If this mutation happens within a gene it can alter its function and so has the potential to cause cancer.

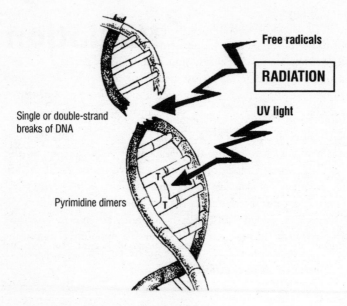

Figure 9 Radiation-induced DNA damage

Skin cancers are one of the most prevalent cancers worldwide and the most common forms of cancer in most pale-skinned peoples. In the UK, for example, there are at least twice as many cases of skin cancer as of the next most common cancers (lung cancer in men and breast cancer in women). Fortunately, most are the *non-melanoma* forms (classified as either basal cell carcinomas or squamous cell carcinomas, depending on the particular layer of the skin in which they form). Non-melanomas have very high rates of cure and are not even included in most rankings of the incidence of different cancer types. The skin cancers that merit particular mention in such statistics are the much less common *malignant melanomas*, a form of pigmented skin cancer.

Almost all of us have many benign tumours of the pigmented cells of our skin, in the form of moles. When a cell within one of these moles sustains further damage to its genes, a change in its growth may be the first sign that it is progressing towards a malignant melanoma. Most health organizations agree on a simple set of rules for spotting such abnormal moles, sometimes referred to as the ABCs of skin cancer: Asymmetry, Border, Colour, Diameter and Elevation (or Evolution). However, as many as half of malignant melanomas may arise as new moles that have already bypassed the controls that limit the growth of our other moles. Malignant melanomas account for only about 10% of all skin cancers, but a significant minority are fatal (one in six to eight cases). Overall, the sun appears to be responsible for about 2,500 deaths in the UK, over 10,000 deaths in the USA and about 55,000 deaths a year worldwide, most of which are due to malignant melanoma.

THE ABCs OF MALIGNANT MELANOMA

A – Asymmetry: one part differs from another
B – Border: irregular, scalloped or poorly defined border
C – Colour: varied from one area to another. Shades of tan and brown or black, sometimes white, red or blue
D – Diameter: while melanomas are usually greater than 6mm in diameter when diagnosed, they can be smaller
E – Elevation: a mole that is raised above the skin is more suspicious; Evolution: if you see your mole change in any way over a period of time, contact your doctor

If you notice a mole that is different from others or which changes, itches or bleeds (even if it is small), you should see a doctor.

Adapted from http://sunsafekids.tripod.com/id2.html

Fortunately, we can take steps to avoid skin cancer. First, we can repel the attack: ultraviolet light is not a particularly powerful form of radiation and so cannot penetrate any substantial barrier. Blocking access to the cells and their DNA will stop its effects. The pigment in our skin, the protein melanin, offers us natural protection. In countries where sunlight is stronger, humans have evolved to be darker-skinned, which protects them from ultraviolet-induced damage as the melanin absorbs and dissipates the ultraviolet energy. As a result, black populations have a very low incidence of skin cancer. Likewise, it seems that long-term exposure to low levels of ultraviolet light, as experienced by

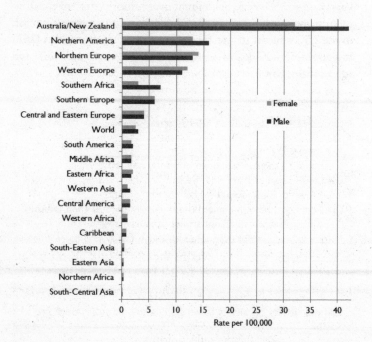

Figure 10 Variation in the incidence of malignant melanoma (2008)

Source: Cancer Research UK, skin cancer statistics report 2013

people who work outdoors in northern Europe, causes a gradual increase in melanin levels and so protects against skin cancer. Of course, we can also avoid this cause of cancer through limiting our exposure to sunlight by covering up and using the many sun-block products available.

Intermittent exposure to high levels of ultraviolet light, such as rapid tanning or sunbathing, is the strongest stimulus of skin cancer. The trouble really comes when pale-skinned people migrate to hot countries such as Australia, which has the world's highest rates of skin cancer and skin cancer-related deaths. The number of deaths in Australia due to skin cancer (about 1,600 a year) is not much over half of that in the UK, but the population of Australia is only 20 million, as compared to about 60 million in the UK. Therefore, we are almost twice as likely to die of skin cancer in New Zealand and Australia than we are in the UK and most other countries in the Northern hemisphere.

It seems that we used to be much better at avoiding exposure to ultraviolet irradiation. Rates of skin cancer have escalated dramatically since the 1970s; there were about four times as many cases and twice as many deaths by the end of the twentieth century than in 1980. Whether this is due to the relaxation in the amount of clothing that has become socially acceptable or the mass emigration to warmer climes for our annual holidays since the 1950s we cannot easily tell. It is striking that the anatomical regions where malignant melanoma are most common varies between men and women and does indeed appear to reflect the way that we expose ourselves to the sun and so where we are most likely to be sunburned. In the UK and many other countries, most cases in men are on the upper body (especially upper back), perhaps because men more often go 'topless' in sunny weather. In women, most cases are on the legs and to a lesser extent the arms, perhaps reflecting the fact that the legs, especially the upper part of the calf, are less chronically exposed to sunlight and so more likely to be burned when sunbathing.

Ultraviolet radiation affects us early in life, through high levels of exposure to sunlight as children and young adults. Extreme and acute exposure, such as sunburn, is particularly associated with an increase in cancer risk. Such events might be more common in the young, when the risks seem less real. This may explain why skin cancer tends to affect us a little earlier than most cancers; almost a third of cases are found in people below 50 years of age. Unfortunately, although few of us can be unaware of the link between ultraviolet light exposure and skin cancer, concern about physical appearance often overrides concern about risk of cancer. The desire to appear tanned leads many people to expose themselves to excessive sunlight, and while the ultraviolet radiation of sunbeds has been linked to skin cancer in much the same way as sunlight, many people nonetheless choose to use them regularly. Because the use of sunbeds is a relatively recent pastime of only a minority of the population, and there is, in general, a time lag of 15 to 30 years between the first carcinogenic events and the appearance of cancer, it will be several more years before we have a really clear idea of the level of cancer sunbeds are causing. Can sunbeds really cause cancer? Cancer Research UK and the International Agency for Research on Cancer agree that use of sunbeds increases your risk of several types of skin cancer – including malignant melanoma. A study in 2014 concluded that almost 10% of malignant melanomas could be attributed to the use of sunbeds. Fortunately, the use of sunbeds by people under the age of 18 is now banned in several European countries and American states.

Any increase in the level of ultraviolet light to which we are exposed, whether through where we live or the changes associated with global warming, could cause an increase in the frequency of skin cancer. However, our risk of skin cancer is primarily linked to whether we allow ourselves to be over-exposed to that light. Our fate, at least in this respect, is very much in our own hands.

Radioactive materials

Other forms of high-energy, ionising radiation are also extremely damaging to DNA, either directly or indirectly causing breaks in our DNA genomes. The mechanism by which all forms of radiation affect our DNA is basically the same: they supply energy to the chemicals in our cells and cause unwanted reactions to occur. The most damaging of these reactions are those that affect our DNA. For ionising radiation, the effect is largely indirect. The energy from the radiation causes the water molecules in our cells to split; the H_2O is separated into H^+ and OH^-. The OH^- molecule is a form of *free radical*, also known as a *reactive oxygen species*.

An atom is neutral when the number of protons (particles with a positive charge) in its nucleus is balanced by an equal number of electrons (particles with a negative charge). However, atoms are only stable when they have an even number of electrons, that is, they exist as pairs. If one is missing, the atom is said to have an *unpaired electron*. Atoms with unpaired electrons find a pair for these electrons by bonding to another atom with an unpaired electron. Free radical molecules have an unpaired electron, and therefore they are very reactive, attacking other molecules in our cells by reacting with them to find a pair for their unpaired electron.

If the molecule with which the free radicals react is DNA, this can result in a break in the DNA strands. Snapping the strands of our DNA cannot be a good thing; if such breaks are not repaired, this will result in death of the cell. The real problem occurs when the cell tries and fails to repair the DNA correctly. DNA breaks occur in normal, healthy cells many times during their lifetime (the breaking and repair of the DNA strands is an essential event in replication, avoiding the DNA becoming tangled), so we have a very effective machinery to repair such breaks, without which the cells would die. This is great for the cell, but it is not so great for us. When DNA is repaired, errors sometimes happen. The more breaks there are, the more repair is needed and the more errors will occur. Since a break in the DNA is repaired by re-joining the two broken ends, a broken end in one chromosome is sometimes re-joined to the broken end from a different chromosome. This is how complicated reorganizations of the chromosomes, frequently seen in most cancers, can occur. It seems that our cells are good at surviving but take rather less care to avoid the possible beginnings of cancer.

Learning from the survivors of the 1945 atomic bombs

Although most of us are unlikely to come into contact with high-energy radiation, many people have suffered its consequences, thanks to its use in weapons and as a source of fuel. Setting aside all ethical issues and the horrors of the events, the studies that have followed the survivors of the Hiroshima and Nagasaki bombs of 1945 have provided an unprecedented insight into the degree to which such massive exposure to radiation can affect the development of cancers.

Those in the immediate vicinity of the blasts inevitably died, either from the explosion itself, the raging firestorms that followed, or the massive cell death and organ failure caused by radiation sickness. However, many people who were within 2.5 kilometres of the blasts did – and indeed still do – survive. Those more than 3 kilometres from the epicentre are regarded as having suffered negligible radiation. Since 1958, a group of about 120,000 individuals who were within 10 kilometres of the centre of the blasts has been followed (over 85% of the 40,000 or so survivors who were less than 20 years old at the time of the bombings were still alive in 1998). By comparing the frequency of various cancers between those who were exposed to the radiation of these bombs and those who were not (for example the many residents of the cities who were not there when the bombs were dropped), researchers have been able to estimate how much this radiation contributed to the cancers that later appeared.

The most recent data available, from 2003, reveals two observations of particular note. First, for most survivors, the increase in the numbers of solid cancer (that is, cancers other than leukaemia) is surprisingly small. Among those who were under the age of 20 at the time of radiation exposure the average risk of developing a solid cancer was only 10–15% greater than those who were not exposed. In other words, where 6 in every 200 people might normally have developed a solid cancer by the age of 65, 7 of every 200 of those exposed to radiation developed such cancers. This large, but single, dose of radiation had a surprisingly small effect on the rate of cancer. However, for the 2–3% of victims nearest to the epicentres of the explosions (less than 1 kilometre away) the level of radiation did result in a much greater increase in incidence of solid cancers. For those aged 30 at the time of the bombs for example, this level of radiation almost doubled their chances of developing cancer by the time they reached the age of 70. The second observation is that the contribution of this radiation to cancers decreases with the increasing age at which individuals were exposed. This is consistent with the radiation causing initial errors in cells, which require further mutational events to occur before cancer arises. Those who were older when they were exposed to the radiation did not have enough time to acquire sufficient additional mutations in the irradiated cells before those people died of other causes.

The situation for leukaemia appears to be worse. The effect on rates of leukaemia was more pronounced and quicker, doubling its incidence from about 16 to 32 per 10,000 people. There does, therefore, appear to be a particularly strong effect of radiation on the cancerous behaviour of blood cells. Interestingly, this is consistent with observations of other populations exposed to radiation, such as after leaks from nuclear power plants or following the Chernobyl disaster in 1986 (when the nuclear core of the oldest nuclear power plant in the Ukraine exploded, resulting in a plume of radioactive fallout that spread across the Soviet Union and Northern Europe). The most commonly accepted explanation for radiation's particular effect on leukaemias is that radiation frequently results in breaks in the DNA strands, and the underlying cause of leukaemia is generally the breaking and incorrect recombination of chromosomes (see chapter 11, p. 125–126 for more on this type of damage in leukaemia). Any event that increases the number of breaks in our DNA – and radiation particularly causes DNA breaks – is likely to increase the frequency of recombination, which can lead to leukaemia. Once this first event has occurred, leukaemia may require fewer subsequent mutations to become fully cancerous than in solid cancers.

Day-to-day exposure

Most of us are only likely to be exposed to high-energy radiation through medical treatments, where levels are not usually high enough to cause significant worry. Unfortunately, for those who first discovered such forms of radiation, the risks were not immediately apparent. Pioneers in the field, such as Marie Curie (who coined the word radioactivity), suffered dire consequences as a result of their work. Marie Curie developed leukaemia and died, aged 66, almost certainly as the result of her exposure to radiation. Tragically, her daughter Irene Curie (somewhat overshadowed by her immensely successful mother, despite the fact that she also was awarded a Nobel Prize in chemistry) developed leukaemia and died aged 57, following a lifetime of research into radioactivity. Clarence Dally, who worked as an assistant to Thomas Edison, was even more unfortunate. Following the discovery of X-rays, Dally routinely exposed himself to this radiation and died from cancer aged only 39, following a long period of suffering and operations. The cause seems to have become clear relatively quickly; the *New York Times* article of 4 October 1904 that reported Dally's death said:

> Clarence M. Dally, electrical engineer, died yesterday at his home, 103 Clinton Street North, East Orange, a martyr to science, the beginning of his illness having been due to his experimental work in connection with the Roentgen rays. For seven years he patiently bore terrible suffering and underwent seven operations, which finally culminated in the amputation of both his arms.

Fortunately, the risks of ionising radiation are now well established and we are rarely subject to damaging levels, but for some one source of radiation is a significant danger. Radon gas, a breakdown product of uranium, is released from certain geological features and can seep into our homes, where, if ventilation is insufficient, it will accumulate. Our risk of exposure depends primarily on where we live: a web search for radon map and the country of your choice will show you where the hot-spots are. Known areas of high radon levels include some parts of Scandinavia and certain areas of North America.

Because the decay products of radon gas, primarily polonium (the radioisotope used to kill the Russian dissident Alexander Litvinenko in London in 2006), are inhaled, they become concentrated in the lungs. These compounds are alpha particle-emitters, a form of radiation that affects cells only over a very short distance. As a result, under these circumstances, the cells that line the lungs are subject to continuous local irradiation. So, exposure to radon gas tends to result in lung cancer. A recent statement from the US Department of Health and Human Services, based on studies in the US, suggested that radon is second only to smoking in causing lung cancers, resulting in 21,000 lung cancer-related deaths each year. Similarly, there may be as many as 20,000 radon-associated cancer deaths per year in Europe. It is unclear what proportion of lung cancers worldwide are attributable to radon exposure, but it is likely to range from as low as 0.5% (in the UK) to most of the 8–10% of cases that are not due to smoking tobacco or exposure to asbestos. It also seems that smoking and radon act synergistically to cause lung cancer (meaning that exposure to both together increases our chances of getting lung cancer significantly more than their two individual effects).

What can we do to protect ourselves from radiation-induced cancer? The bottom line is, avoid the radiation. This can be quite easily achieved for sunlight; it is generally our choice whether we expose ourselves to excessive ultraviolet radiation. The situation for ionising radiation is more difficult. Awareness of the risks and regional concentrations of radon gas make it possible to design our homes to reduce risk of exposure. In the medical world, although screening and treatment for cancer itself mean we might be exposed to radiation, new therapies are being developed that might eventually allow us to avoid this exposure altogether. Other than this, the only other source of radiation we are likely to be exposed to is through nuclear weapons or nuclear power and this must be dealt with by our broader society.

Summary

Radiation from sunlight or from radioactive sources is a powerful DNA damaging force. Hence, any substantial exposure to radiation can damage DNA and so result in mutations in our DNA that has the potential to lead to cancer. For most of us, the only radiation we are at a high risk of being exposed to is the UV radiation of sunlight or sunbeds. It is not surprising then that those who fail to heed advice to avoid exposure to strong UV light are at a much greater risk of skin cancer. Most skin cancers are of the non-pigmented cells, which are rarely malignant and are relatively easy to remove. However, cancer of pigmented skin cells, malignant melanoma, is one of the most aggressive cancers, often resulting in death. For the unfortunate people who are exposed to strong radiation of other types the most immediate effect is to induce breaks in the DNA strands, which dramatically increases their risk of developing leukaemia. However, as the survivors of the World War II nuclear attacks in Japan illustrate, this type of radiation is also quite non-specific, eventually leading to a wide range of cancer types.

8
Catching cancer

The examples discussed so far show how cancer is caused by physical insults that damage our DNA and result in mutations in our genes. However, it is also possible to 'catch' cancer, or, to be more precise, catch the predisposition to develop cancer. Like most infectious diseases, the microscopic organisms involved are either viruses or bacteria.

Table 2 Main micro-organisms that play a role in cancer

Micro-organism	Types of cancer	Number of cancers worldwide per year	Estimated number of cancer deaths worldwide per year
Helicobacter pylori (*H. pylori*) bacterium	Stomach cancer	930,000	700,000
Hepatitis viruses (HBV/HCV)	Liver cancer	450,000	450,000
Human Papilloma Virus (HPV)	Cervical cancer	490,000	235,000
Epstein-Barr Virus (EBV)	Nasopharyngeal cancer (upper part of throat) and lymphoma	100,000	50,000
Human Immunodeficiency Virus (HIV)	Kaposi's sarcoma and other rarer tumours	57,000*	52,000*

* This estimate is for Africa only, since this is where AIDS is most prevalent. Cancer is a major problem for those infected with HIV elsewhere in the world but the numbers are much smaller.

Appendix 3 contains a more detailed description of the mechanisms by which these infectious agents can cause cancer.

To a large extent, infectious agents do not act like carcinogens (see chapter 6). Rather than causing damage to our own genes, these viruses often carry their own cancer-initiating genes into the cell, providing a first step towards cancer. Once a cell is infected, the virus is inherited by daughter cells as that cell divides. The effect of the viral genes varies depending upon the type of virus but often involves increased proliferation of the cell. The more that cells proliferate the more opportunity there is for mutations to occur, hence these virally infected cells become more prone to acquire mutations and so eventually become fully cancerous. Fortunately, only four types of virus and one type of bacterium are implicated in any significant number of cancers.

Viruses and cancer

In most countries, the Epstein-Barr virus causes proliferation of lymphocytes (the white blood cells that act as the main frontline of our immune response) in about half of infected teenagers. Most commonly, this leads to the disease variously known as glandular fever or mono (infectious mononucleosis), but in a large region of Africa, Epstein-Barr virus infection is associated with a cancer called Burkitt's lymphoma. Named after Denis Burkitt, it is the most common children's tumour seen in central Africa (it was from a sample of one such tumour that Anthony Epstein and Yvonne Barr first isolated the virus in 1964).

In Southeast Asia, the same virus is associated with a tumour of a different type of cell, resulting in nasopharyngeal cancer, a highly disfiguring cancer of the nose and mouth. The reason these severe consequences are restricted to Africa and Southeast Asia appears to be associated with immune suppression. In Africa, co-infection with the malarial parasite weakens the body's defences and allows the Epstein-Barr virus to have a dramatic effect on the cells it infects. The explanation why it leads to such a particular cancer in Asia remains unclear. The result is that the

Epstein–Barr virus is responsible for over 100,000 cancers per year worldwide.

Although more than 300 million people worldwide are infected by the hepatitis B or C viruses (mostly in parts of Africa, China and Southeast Asia), in most of us, infection with either virus normally results in a relatively mild and often curable disease, hepatitis. This is the inflammation of the liver, which is due largely to the immune system's response to the viral infection. However, infection with a hepatitis virus also carries the risk of cancer of the liver, resulting in about 600,000 cases per year. Liver cancer is the sixth most common cancer worldwide, but it is very often fatal. Almost all of those diagnosed with liver cancer will die from the disease, making it third in the list for cancer-related deaths. What makes liver cancer of particular concern is that it is heavily biased towards less developed countries, but it could be, to a large extent, avoided through education and vaccination.

Whether in parts of Asia, where the risk of developing liver cancer can approach one in 1,000, or Europe and North America, where the risk is less than one in 10,000, more than 3 out of 4 cases of liver cancer appear to be directly linked to infection by either the hepatitis B or hepatitis C virus. So why does the virus only cause cancer in a minority of infected individuals? The answer appears to be that the cancer is a consequence of chronic infection over many years. Hence, cancer results primarily when infection first occurred in childhood, a situation more common in less developed countries. Fortunately, current vaccines against hepatitis B and C viruses are quite effective and the result of vaccination programmes in Taiwan and South Korea are very encouraging, resulting in a dramatic decrease in liver cancer incidence. The virus is generally spread either through sexual intercourse or via contaminated blood. Improved screening of blood products and public education programmes to avoid infection mean that liver cancer rates are expected to fall substantially as the fruits of these public health measures become apparent.

For those living in developed counties, the virus of most concern with respect to cancer is likely to be Human Papilloma Virus (HPV), which is associated with most cases of cervical cancer. Papilloma viruses are generally associated with benign warts, but they are also responsible for almost 500,000 cases of cervical cancer each year, making them the most common cancer-causing infectious agents, just ahead of the hepatitis viruses. Cervical cancer occurs relatively early in life, peaking in women between the ages of 25 and 30. In some countries (including the UK), it is the most common cancer in women under 35. The young age at which this cancer appears is very likely to be because the virus elicits many of the changes necessary for cancer to form, reducing the number of genes that need to become mutated. The result is a lag time of only 10 to 20 years from infection to cancer diagnosis.

There are more than 100 sub-types of HPV, but HPV 16 and HPV 18 are found in over 99% of cervical cancers. Other sub-types of HPV cause genital warts, but these do not carry an increased risk of cervical cancer. Between 40–80% of women are estimated to become infected with HPV (depending on the country in which they live), but in most the infections are cleared within a few years. Like smoking and lung cancer, there seems to be a simple way to avoid this type of cancer: abstain from sexual intercourse. Having few sexual partners, practising protected sex and following a monogamous lifestyle are all believed to reduce the risk of cervical cancer. This disease is rarely found in those who are celibate; nuns have a much-reduced frequency of this cancer (although the number of nuns available for study – or indeed any women who have abstained from sexual activity for their whole lives – is too small to draw definitive conclusions about the protective effects of abstinence).

The association between age and cervical cancer cases and deaths is confused by geographical differences and dramatic changes in sexual activity and the prevalence of HPV over time.

For example, British women born at the end of the nineteenth century and around 1920 suffer a higher cervical cancer mortality rate than women born at other times early in the twentieth century. The explanation seems to lie in the fact that women born at these times would have been in their 20s during the world wars and so experienced the more liberal sexual behaviour of those periods.

Although survival rates have improved dramatically over the past 30 years, in the UK almost 40% of women with cervical cancer do not survive their disease more than 10 years after their diagnosis. The figures are better in the young; women below the age of 40 have a survival rate about double that of those diagnosed in their 60s and 70s. However, the outlook for this particular cancer looks very positive, due to the development of an effective vaccine (Gardasil) against the main causative agent, HPV. Since its licensing in 2007, the health services of over 80 countries have instigated vaccination programmes against HPV infection for girls before they become sexually active. We must hope this will save many of these young women from the severe, and sometimes fatal, consequences of cervical cancer.

Unlike the many steps required for individual mutations to lead to the initiation of cancer, the activity of most of these viruses causes cancer to arise rather rapidly. One explanation is the power of the oncogenes they carry. The E6 and E7 genes of HPV, for example, code for proteins that can inactivate both the Rb and P53 tumour suppressors (described in chapters 2 and 3 and Appendix 1 p.185–188). This may explain why virally induced cancers are more often seen in younger people. On the positive side, because viruses are genuinely alien invaders, our immune system normally eradicates them before they can lead to cancer. It is often only when they are associated with suppression of the immune system that they have the opportunity to persist long enough for the cancer to develop. This explains why the fourth virus associated with cancer predisposition, HIV, is so difficult to deal with. The effects of HIV on the immune system facilitate the growth of cancers. Not only does the body fail to fight against other viral infections it is also less able to detect and eradicate tumour cells.

For pet lovers, I should point out that we have long known that viruses are a relatively common cause of cancer in domestic animals such as cats, dogs and chickens. For example, the feline leukaemia virus is one of the leading causes of death in cats. We are fortunate that the same types of virus do not generally infect the human population.

Bacteria and cancer

Most, possibly all, cases of stomach cancer involve infection by the bacterium *Helicobacter pylori* (*H. pylori*). This bacterium was initially found in 1982, in patients with gastritis, an inflammation of the stomach lining, which precedes the occurrence of stomach ulcers. The Australian physician and Nobel Prize winner, Barry Marshall, revolutionized our understanding of the cause of this inflammation when he chose to swallow a culture of *H. pylori* – and he got gastritis! However, like the Epstein–Barr and hepatitis viruses, while half the world's population is infected with *H. pylori*, only a small proportion gets stomach cancer. It is not yet clear why this is, but it is likely to reflect the particular sub-type of the bacterium, aspects of our diet and possibly our individual immune response to the infection.

The role of *H. pylori* infection in cancer is thought to be indirect: the bacteria cause inflammation due to the toxins they release and the inflammation is thought to promote the initiation of cancer. *H. pylori* infection, and therefore stomach cancer, is more prevalent in some regions (such as the Far East, Eastern Europe, Polynesia and South America) than others. Remarkably, there is evidence to suggest that treating *H. pylori* infections with a simple course of antibiotics virtually eradicates the possibility of stomach cancer, making this one of the most 'curable' causes of cancer. Yet stomach cancer remains second only to lung cancer as a cause of death worldwide (about 700,000 deaths per year).

Avoidable cancers?

Most of the cancer-causing agents described in these chapters could be of little consequence to us. We simply need to avoid them. Is this such a tall order? The monks of Mount Athos would probably say not. If we were to cut red meat from our diet, stop smoking and steer clear of unprotected sex, we would avoid many of the major cancer-causing agents. However, exposure to asbestos or becoming infected with viruses such as hepatitis B or the bacterium *H. pylori* is unlikely to be within our control. Many of these risks could, however, be dealt with much more effectively by our broader societies. Asbestos use could be abolished worldwide, we could be vaccinated against HPV and other viruses and we could treat *H. pylori* infections. The only real barriers are money and the commitment of our society.

Many of these potentially avoidable cancers are largely restricted to less economically developed countries, due in part to the export of the causes of cancer by the wealthy West in pursuit of even greater wealth. So how many cancers are truly unavoidable? If we take the number of cases in the country with the minimum rate for each type of cancer as the maximum likely unavoidable rate, it would appear that only about 30% of cancers (most of these in women, see chapter 9) would occur in the absence of modern toxins, such as cigarette smoke. At a conservative estimate, a careful lifestyle and ambitious public health schemes could reduce worldwide cancer cases from the current level of around 10 million a year by more than half.

But this still leaves a lot of unavoidable cancers.

Summary

Cancer is not generally thought of as a disease that you can 'catch'. This is largely because, for those who live in developed countries, cancer is very rarely caused by infectious agents. Most infectious sources of cancer are viruses, which affect people in developing countries where their bodies are also weakened by other factors. In the West, cervical cancer and gastric cancer are the only major types of cancer with a strong association with infections. Both of these are treatable, via vaccination or antibiotics respectively, and so are among the cancers that are in decline in the West. It is unfortunate that such public health interventions are not currently available for most people in poorer countries where infection-driven cancers are most prevalent.

Part 3
Who gets cancer?

9

We are all different

Although for most of us, it is our exposure to carcinogens that determines our risk of developing cancer, the same exposure does not affect everyone in the same way. Our physiology, the precise nature and state of our bodies that is largely a reflection of our genetic make-up, affects our responses. However, different responses to carcinogens can also be due to other aspects of our body's functions, such as hormonal variations or the changes that occur as we move from childhood into adulthood.

Protection and vulnerability

In many ways, the genes we inherit from our parents provide us with a template for our future lives. They dictate our sex, our blood group and our eye colour and have a significant influence on our likelihood of becoming ill. Our genes determine many aspects of our bodies' functions that affect how we respond to disease-causing events in our environment, for example why some people smoke heavily all their lives and never develop cancer, while some light smokers do. Presently, we understand little of what underlies such variation but it is clear that many genes contribute to our susceptibility to the effects of carcinogens.

Although we all have the same basic set of genes, such as the genes that code for our hair colour or control of our cell cycle, the precise gene sequence has changed during human evolution, resulting in many, many different versions of each gene scattered amongst the human population. The reason we all look different and we all have subtly different metabolisms is that we each have slightly different versions of each gene. This variation in gene sequences explains why, if one of our siblings develops a cancer, our probability of developing that same cancer is higher than would be expected in the general population. In breast cancer, for example, the greatest risk factor is having another family member with the same disease. Members of the same family have a similar susceptibility to cancer because siblings inherit their genes from the same parents, so share more identical genes with each other than they do with people in the general population. So members of the same family will have a more similar susceptibility to the same carcinogenic events than would two unrelated individuals.

The link between our genes and our chances of developing disease is most striking in identical twins, in whom every gene is identical. If the small variations in the sequence of our genes were irrelevant and cancer arose simply due to random mutations in key genes, the chances of identical twins suffering the same coincidence of events would be no greater than for any other siblings. However, large studies, including thousands of twins, show that an identical twin of someone who develops colon, stomach, breast or prostate cancer is much more likely to develop the same cancer. For example, in one study, an identical twin of someone who had stomach cancer was 10 times more likely to develop stomach cancer than an identical twin of someone who did not have stomach cancer. For each twin, whether they develop cancer is still a matter of chance, requiring the random genetic damage induced by carcinogens to hit six or more key genes in the same cell. However, such studies show that variations in the precise sequence of the genes we carry result in the variations we see in our susceptibility to these mutations or their consequences, so certain people are less protected against particular cancers than are others.

Which of the genes that vary among us affect our risk of developing a cancer? You can probably make a pretty good guess; it is variations in any gene in any of the processes that protect us against cancer. This includes the genes that code for proteins important in the DNA repair machinery, the cell cycle checkpoints or the systems that protect us against carcinogens. Some versions of these genes may be good, improving the machinery that protects us from cancer, and others may be bad, making us more prone to cancer. For some cancers, the explanation can be simple, such as carrying a defective gene for alcohol breakdown (chapter 6, p. 73). For skin cancer, some people – red-haired people, for example – are more sensitive to the damaging effects of ultraviolet radiation. Instead of tanning (the process by which melanocytes, the pigmented skin cells, produce melanin to absorb and diffuse the ultraviolet energy), these people just burn. People with red hair often possess a different version of the gene that makes the cellular receptor needed to tell melanocytes to make melanin. This version of the gene makes a less effective receptor, so the melanocytes make very little melanin in response to stimulation by ultraviolet light.

These effects, and other even weaker effects due to the variations among our individual genomes, are very hard to identify, since their association with cancer is so subtle. However, as we become better at analysing a person's entire genome, we are better able to identify specific gene sequences that affect their chances of developing cancer or even predict how they might respond to therapy. With this information, we should eventually be able to tailor treatments better to the individual patient, providing a route to improved therapy (chapter 13, p. 163–166).

The trouble with hormones

For some cancers, it seems that our particular genes and our exposure to carcinogens are not the only risk factors. This is particularly true of those cancers primarily restricted to women and may partly explain why breast cancer is so prevalent. Worldwide, the number of people suffering from breast cancer is second only to lung cancer, but among women it is by far the most common cancer. In the West, rates of breast cancer in women are twice that of lung cancer.

THE STATISTICS OF BREAST CANCER

The incidence of breast cancer has risen rapidly in developed countries since the 1970s. Because our genes do not alter that rapidly, we must assume this increase is due to changes in our environment. Globally, each year over 1.5 million women are diagnosed with breast cancer, accounting for one in four of all female cancers. In the UK, cases of breast cancer outnumber the next three most common types of cancer in women (bowel, lung, uterus) combined. If we remove lung cancer from the equation (not smoking would largely achieve this), breast cancer would be responsible for almost 20% of cancer-related deaths in women. About one in eight UK women will develop breast cancer and about one in five of them will not survive their cancer beyond ten years after diagnosis, dying at a younger age than for most other types of cancer. Unlike most other cancers, we cannot attribute these figures to any readily identified carcinogens. For many women, breast cancer seems to be an entirely unavoidable disease. Fortunately, early diagnosis and improved treatments mean that survival rates have improved dramatically. In the 1970s, two out of five women could expect to survive their disease for at least ten years after diagnosis. In 2010, this number had risen to almost four out of five patients. This suggests that today most women will survive breast cancer long term.

Of all types of cancer, breast cancer is the most frequently described form of cancer in historical records, known even before the advent of modern carcinogens. This is just one piece

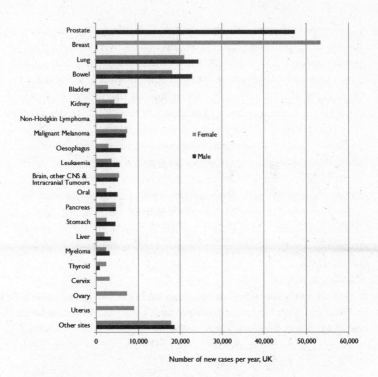

Figure 11 The most common cancers in men and women in the UK Excludes non-melanoma skin cancer.

Source: Cancer Research UK

of evidence that suggests that events within the body itself are a driving force for these cancers. It is clear that some level of risk and the early onset of this cancer may relate to the special nature of female biology. I have already mentioned the observation that nuns have a reduced risk of cervical cancer. Current statistics also strongly suggest that a nun's lifestyle increases her risk of developing breast cancer, because breast cancer is, in part, an unfortunate side effect of women's hormonal systems.

Women's bodies function in much the same way that they always have, priming them for ovulation once a month, for up to 30 to 40 years. Every month, the ovaries produce the hormones oestrogen and progesterone, which cause the lining of the uterus to thicken and stimulate the milk ducts of the breast. In short, women undergo a monthly cycle of hormonal surges designed to trigger an increase in cellular proliferation and other changes in breast tissue. In particular, oestrogen stimulates growth of the milk ducts; cancer of this particular tissue is the most common form of breast cancer. However, the increase in proliferation in breast tissue is not very great and there may be other reasons why these hormonal surges favour the development of breast cancer. There is evidence, for example, that the Cyp enzymes, which in some circumstances cause environmental toxins to become carcinogenic (chapter 6, p. 72), can likewise convert oestrogen into a carcinogen.

Since the purpose of these cycles of hormone production is to ready a woman for pregnancy, childbirth and breastfeeding, the body shuts the cycles down once that end is achieved. Once a woman is pregnant, the monthly bursts of sex hormones stop, as does the consequent cell proliferation. After nine months, breastfeeding continues to subdue the hormones that stimulate cellular proliferation in the breast and uterus, by inducing the production of a hormone, prolactin, which inhibits ovulation and the associated monthly bursts of oestrogen and progesterone. For this reason, earlier and more frequent pregnancies will reduce the amount of time during a woman's life in which she is subject to hormonal surges, as will the frequency and length of breastfeeding. It has been estimated that a woman reduces her life-time risk of developing breast cancer by 7% for each live birth and an additional 4% for every year that she breastfeeds. A rough calculation shows that a woman who does not give birth to children will go through as many as 400 rounds of sex hormone production during her lifetime, whereas a woman who has a large family, of perhaps 6 children, whom she breastfeeds for an average of 18 to 24 months each, would lose around 200 of these cycles, a reduction of 50%, with a consequent 70% reduction in her risk of developing breast cancer. The pattern seen in most economically developed countries, of delaying first pregnancies to a later age and breastfeeding for only a few weeks or months, therefore results in increased risk. In the UK the incidence of breast cancer will reflect an average live birth rate of approximately two and an average breast feeding period of about six months each, resulting in an 18% reduction in risk.

One change to the modern woman's lifestyle in recent decades is the use of hormonal treatments such as the contraceptive pill and hormone replacement therapies (HRT). These treatments generally include a combination of oestrogen and progesterone or one of these alone, hormones that not only regulate the female reproductive organs but also play a role in some cancers of these tissues.

The contraceptive pill has been shown to result in a small increase the risk of breast cancer, largely due to its oestrogen content. Some studies have also associated the use of oral contraceptives with an increased risk of cervical cancer, but the link could be due to the fact that women who take the pill are less likely to use barrier contraceptives and are therefore more likely to acquire an HPV infection, a primary cause of cervical cancer (chapter 8, p. 93–94). However, research suggests oral contraceptives bring a decreased risk of cancer of the uterus, ovaries and colon. The form of pill generally prescribed in the UK is low in oestrogen, so its overall effect on cancer risk is likely to be small.

The risks associated with HRT are more serious and vary according to the specific type of therapy and the circumstances of the women concerned. Although some smaller research reports (which have been highlighted in the popular press) did not find any increase in cancer risk, many other studies involving many millions of women show that these drugs do significantly increase the risk of cancer. Overall, recent studies suggest that some of the most commonly used HRT regimes more than double the risk of breast cancer. This might not seem so bad if a cancer were rare, but breast cancer is not a rare disease. This raises the risk of developing breast cancer during the period that HRT might be taken (50–70 years of age) from about one in twelve to one in six women. This doubled risk is only seen using combined oestrogen-progesterone treatments. Oestrogen or tibolone (a synthetic drug with actions similar to both oestrogen and progesterone) alone raise the risk to about one in eight women developing breast cancer. However, in women who still retain their uterus, oestrogen-only HRT also increases the risk of endometrial cancer (a cancer of the uterus) so in these women the overall increased risk of any cancer is about the same as the combined oestrogen plus progesterone form of HRT (half of these are endometrial cancers, which have a similar survival rate to breast cancer). However, many women take HRT after a hysterectomy (removal of the uterus), which removes any risk of endometrial cancer. Therefore, unsurprisingly, oestrogen-only HRT does carry a significantly lower risk in women who have had a hysterectomy. Oestrogen-only HRT also carries an increased risk of ovarian cancer (which has a relatively poor prognosis), but this is likely to result in very few cases compared to the number of breast or endometrial cancer.

Although the net effect of HRT appears to be an increase in cancer risk, this is offset by some reduction in the risk of developing cancer of the colon or rectum, although the data here is less clear. Some recent studies also found a possible 40–60% reduced mortality rate in those women who developed colon cancer. Overall, therefore, HRT might reduce the colon cancer risk from about 5 women per 100 to about 3 women per 100, and the death risk from colon cancer by about 1 in 100. Clearly, even if these reports prove to be correct, these positive side effects are a long way from balancing increased risk of breast or endometrial cancer.

The effects of both the contraceptive pill and HRT are proportional to the length of time they are taken. And any increased risk of cancer is lost after the treatment ceases, almost disappearing within one year of stopping HRT and within ten years of stopping the contraceptive pill. Also, the risk declines the longer after menopause a woman waits before beginning HRT treatment, although even starting combined oestrogen plus progesterone HRT five years after menopause, the breast cancer risk would still be raised by about 50%.

The obvious benefits of these drugs should not be dismissed, but in recent years the associated risks have begun to influence their use. For this reason, use of HRT was halved following the first substantial reports of its associated risks. Indeed, a drop in the number of breast cancer cases being recorded in countries such as the USA has been attributed by some to this decreased use of HRT. Taking all the risks and benefits of these treatments into account, determining when the benefits outweigh the risks remains a very personal decision.

Breast tissue is not immune from other environmental risk factors: diet, obesity and alcohol consumption all increase the risk of breast cancer. The rapid increase in breast cancer in Western countries since the 1980s also suggests as yet unidentified carcinogenic risk factors. In addition, your risk of breast cancer is strongly affected by whether another member of your family has had this disease. This tells us that the variations in our genes also play a major role in determining whether we will develop breast cancer.

Looking on the bright side, the unusual hormone dependence of breast cancers has provided some of the best targets for new treatments, with the result that breast cancer leads the way in new biological therapies (see chapter 13).

Men have hormones too

Women are particularly unfortunate in being prone to cancers that reflect the hormonal regulation of their reproductive organs. Since men lack both those organs and the associated hormonal cycles, do they escape such risks? They do not: although men do not possess breasts of the same mass and physiology as women's, nonetheless, they can suffer from breast cancer, although the numbers are tiny compared to women (300 men a year are diagnosed in the UK, compared to about 125 women each day).

However, the male testes are, like the reproductive organs in women, a site of hormone-dependent proliferation. Testicular cancer appears earlier in life than most cancers, with a peak incidence, for some types, between the ages of 15 and 40. Despite an, as yet unexplained, increasing rate, especially in developed countries and particularly among white Caucasians, testicular cancer is not common; it accounts for only about 1% of male cancers and is rarely fatal. Like breast cancer, the affected organ is frequently removed, and, with radiotherapy and/or chemotherapy treatment, current survival rates can be as high as 98%. This has not always been so; before the introduction of modern chemotherapeutic agents in the 1970s (or later in some countries) survival rates were less than 70%. My father was one of many unfortunate men who died young of testicular cancer, before these developments. The curability of testicular cancer is testament to the progress we have made in cancer treatment.

The most common cancer of elderly men occurs in the prostate. Although it is the fifth most common cancer worldwide, much less common than lung, colorectal and stomach cancer in men, prostate is by far the most common cancer of men in the West, accounting for about one in four cancers and second only to lung cancer in cancer-related deaths. It seems likely that carcinogens play a central role in its development but, like the

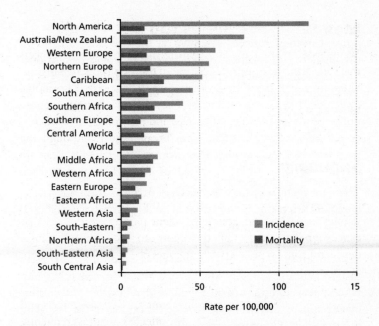

Figure 12 Worldwide incidence of prostate cancer

Note: survival is much better in developed countries such that the level of mortality is relatively constant across the globe.

Source: Cancer Research UK

cancers specific to women, hormones also play a significant part in this male-specific cancer. The prostate is where the fluid of the semen is produced and its growth is regulated by the male sex hormone, testosterone (an androgen; from the Greek 'man maker'). Not surprisingly, testosterone also seems to be important to the survival of prostate cancer cells although, unlike the hormonally dependent cancers of women, prostate cancer is very much a cancer of the old. Other than not ageing, there appears to be little we can do to avoid it. This is somewhat surprising, since it seems the environment significantly influences the development of these cancers, as shown by the dramatic variation in the incidence of prostate cancer, both geographically and over time: in some Western countries, numbers have trebled since 1975. Unfortunately, we have yet to determine what is causing these variations.

Summary

There are many ways in which each of us differs from our neighbours and this includes differences in our likelihood of developing cancer. Genetic differences between individuals not only make us look different to one another, but also make our cells more or less resistant to DNA damage and its effects. It is these differences that, in part, explain why some people never get cancer, despite what appears to be a particularly unhealthy lifestyle, while others live exemplary lifestyles, but develop cancer never-the-less. The most striking difference between individuals is our sex and the factors associated with male or female physiology. What is less intuitive is that it is the very 'hormonal' nature of our reproductive organs that makes them so prone to cancer. Cancers of the sexual organs are often driven by the same hormones that regulate the normal growth and behaviour of the organs themselves.

10
Inheriting cancer

For most of us, our chances of developing cancer depend on the extent to which we are exposed to carcinogens and subtle variations in our genetic makeup. The cancers that appear are sporadic, occurring in an almost random way, afflicting one person in the crowd as a consequence of an unfortunate coincidence of events. However, for some people, the situation is far worse, because they have inherited a defective copy of one key gene, a tumour suppressor gene (chapter 2, p. 25), leading to a strong predisposition to develop cancer.

Although such people are comparatively rare, and the vast majority of cancers are predominantly due to environmental carcinogens, inheritance of mutations in many different genes results in a predisposition to cancer. These defects do not cause small changes in our risk of developing cancer as is seen for the genetic variation between individuals as described in the previous chapter. Each of the genes described here that is occasionally inherited in a mutant form tends to give rise to a particular type of cancer and the increase in risk is enormous, making it highly likely or in some cases, almost certain, that cancer will occur. Most people with these disorders carry the mutant gene in all of the cells of their body, because they inherited that mutated gene from their parents. With respect to cancer, the gene defect results in a relatively minor cellular defect in all cells, which is one step in the cancer-forming process. Since this is only one of the many steps needed for a cancer to develop, these cells generally behave normally, so it sounds like the situation for these people is not so dire.

However, stop to compare this with the rest of us, in whom the first event happens in one, unfortunate cell; for a cancer to occur, a second event must coincidentally occur in that same cell. Clearly, in a person who inherits a defective gene, the odds of one cell acquiring two mutations are far higher than for the rest of us. All their cells have the first mutation, so no matter which cell of the body gets the next mutation, that cell will now have taken two steps towards cancer. Think of our cells as millions of little time bombs: for one to explode, its safety catch must be released and then its fuse must be triggered. If each of these is a one-in-a-million event, the chances of both happening together are vanishingly small, but if all the bombs already have the safety catch released, activating the fuse in any one of them will cause an explosion. Like the bomb with its safety catch released and its fuse triggered, once a cell has sustained two of the events leading towards cancer, its continued march in that direction sometimes becomes unstoppable. Most of those who inherit such predispositions (all the cells having the safety catch released) *will* get cancer, often at a relatively young age.

DOMINANT AND RECESSIVE MUTATIONS IN CANCER

We have two copies of every gene, one inherited from each of our parents. In many cases, if one copy of a gene is damaged by mutation, the cell can continue to function normally, because the second copy remains fully functional. This type of event is a recessive mutation. The consequences of a defect in such a gene are only seen if both copies of the gene are damaged. The alternative situation is when damage to only one copy of a gene results in a detrimental change in the cell or the body. In such a case this normally means that the mutation has led to increased or abnormal activity of the protein that the gene encodes, rather than its inactivation. This kind of mutation is referred to as dominant, where the mutated gene is dominant over the normal gene.

When we inherit a recessive mutation for a particular disease (such as cystic fibrosis, sickle cell anaemia and various muscular dystrophies) all of our cells will still contain one good copy of the gene and we would not exhibit symptoms of that disease, even if

DOMINANT AND RECESSIVE MUTATIONS IN CANCER (*Cont.*)

the good copy of the gene subsequently becomes damaged in a few cells. However, if the mutation predisposes to cancer, the situation is somewhat different. If we inherit one defective copy of the gene and any one cell acquires a damaging mutation in the good copy of the gene, this makes that cell very likely to progress to becoming cancerous.

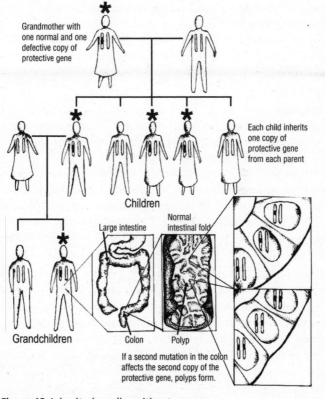

Grandmother with one normal and one defective copy of protective gene

Each child inherits one copy of protective gene from each parent

Children

Grandchildren

Large intestine

Normal intestinal fold

Colon   Polyp

If a second mutation in the colon affects the second copy of the protective gene, polyps form.

Figure 13 Inherited predisposition to cancer

DOMINANT AND RECESSIVE MUTATIONS IN CANCER (*Cont.*)

In Figure 13, the grandmother carries one defective copy (black) and one normal copy (white) of a gene that is important to protect from cancer. Each child of these grandparents inherits one copy of this gene from each parent; there is therefore a 50/50 chance of each child inheriting the defective copy. In the final generation shown, each child also has a 50/50 chance of inheriting the defective copy. All the individuals that carry the defective gene (marked with an asterisk) have an increased risk, so that, eventually, most would develop cancer.

Cancer only occurs if both copies of the gene are defective. Therefore the behaviour of the vast majority of cells in these individuals is completely normal. But if the remaining good copy of the gene becomes damaged or replaced by the bad copy in any single cell, then cancer begins, and, as for most of the syndromes described in this chapter, full-blown cancer will certainly ensue. All of the cells of the cancer will be descended from that one unfortunate cell and will carry two defective copies of the gene.

In most cases these mutations originally appear as if from nowhere in one member of a family. The parents will be as healthy as any of us, but as their sperm and egg cells are made, genes become mutated. During their formation, egg and sperm cells are especially prone to mutations. The egg is the result of about twenty-two cell divisions, all made in five months of foetal development. Because men produce a vast number of sperm in their lives, by the time they form mature sperm, these cells have undergone many more cell divisions than the egg. The first sperm that are produced in puberty are the result of as many as 265 divisions; in a man aged 50 they will have undergone up to 850 cell divisions. Since more cell divisions provide the opportunity for more mutations to arise, mutations are more often inherited from one's father than from one's mother, so-called *paternal bias*.

Once a defect occurs in one founding member of a family, it can be inherited through several generations. Some members of each generation may be lucky and avoid inheriting the defective gene, but their siblings may be less fortunate and share the same defect as their parents. In general, for cancer, the inheritance takes a dominant form, which means that only one parent needs to have the defective gene for it to cause the syndrome in some of their children (and on average 50% of their offspring will inherit the defective gene).

Although these various inherited predispositions are generally described as rare, all the different rare cancer predisposition syndromes represent a very significant health issue when added together. Most of us are lucky enough to have just a one in three chance of developing cancer, even considering all the carcinogens we encounter. People with a genetic predisposition represent a tiny proportion of the world's population, but, because of the power of these mutations in weakening their cells' defences against cancer, they represent as many as 5–10% of the world's cancer sufferers, perhaps 500,000 cancer deaths a year. Cancers that arise through inherited predisposition may be rare by comparison to the sporadic cancers that threaten to kill most of us, but they are not insignificant.

These cancer predisposition syndromes come in many forms, depending on the specific gene that is defective. When the gene has a role in a particular cell type, a restricted range of cancers will occur. If the gene plays a central role in many different cell types, the predisposition may include many forms of cancer. This latter type is actually very unusual. The only major example of such a general cancer predisposition syndrome was first described in 1982, by Frederick Pei Li and Joseph F. Fraumeni (hence called Li-Fraumeni syndrome), and has still been identified in only a few hundred families worldwide. Because those who suffer from Li-Fraumeni syndrome inherit a defective copy of their P53 gene, a key protector against cancer in all of our cells (chapter 3, p. 37, appendix 1 p185–188), they develop a wide range of cancers, often during childhood.

Table 3 Familial cancer syndromes

Syndrome	Genes affected	Frequency in the population	Cancer predisposition
Li-Fraumeni	P53	*	Most organs
Hereditary breast cancer	BRCA1 & 2	1/150–800	Breast and ovary (some association with prostate cancer)
Hereditary non-polyposis colon cancer	Mismatch repair genes	1/3,000	Bowel (colorectal) (some association with endometrial cancer)
Familial adenomatous polyposis	APC	1/10,000	Colorectal (some association with bone cancer)
Retinoblastoma	Rb	1/20,000	Retina
Neurofibromatosis	NF1/NF2	1/3000	Skin (neurofibromas), cancers of the nervous system
Xeroderma pigmentosa	Nucleotide Excision Repair pathway genes	1/250,000	Skin (some association with cancers of brain, lung, stomach, breast, uterus, testes and leukaemias)
Ataxia telangiectasia	Double-strand break repair	1/300,000	Blood (lymphoblastic) and breast. Less often skin, stomach, pancreas, ovary and brain

* Li-Fraumeni syndrome has only been reported in a few hundred families world-wide, so no accurate estimate of its frequency is available. Further details about some of these syndromes are available in Appendix 4.

Inheriting colon cancer

Of all the syndromes that predispose to cancer in a specific tissue, those that increase the risk of cancers of the digestive system are the most common. About 5% of colon cancers are hereditary. This means that, in the USA, about 7,500 colon cancers arise each year as a result of inheritance of a gene mutation. These can be grouped based on the number of *polyps* that sufferers develop. Polyps are small, benign, finger-like projections from the lining of the gut, a type of *adenoma* (benign tumour of epithelial or glandular origin). People who develop very large numbers of polyps suffer from a syndrome known as familial adenomatous polyposis coli, while those who develop very few polyps have a syndrome known as hereditary non-polyposis colon cancer. Not only are these amongst the most prevalent of cancer-predisposing syndromes, they are amongst the most common of all inherited diseases.

Familial adenomatous polyposis was originally identified by Eldon J. Gardner in the early 1950s, in a large Utah family brought to his attention by a medical student he was teaching. The student had noticed that a family in his neighbourhood suffered a surprisingly high incidence of cancer. Fortunately, this family was, as Gardner wrote, 'cooperative in clinical investigations', and was therefore studied at length. Among the cancers that arose in this family, many were carcinomas of the digestive tract, which appeared in about half of this large family of 51 people by the end of Gardner's study. It soon became evident that the appearance of full-blown colon cancer was preceded by the appearance of hundreds or thousands of benign polyps leading to the term polyposis (many polyps) being adopted to describe the disease. As we now know to be the case in most families with this syndrome, both large numbers of adenomatous polyps and subsequent full-blown colorectal cancer arise in all the individuals (about half the family members) who inherit the defective gene.

The second major colon cancer syndrome is hereditary non-polyposis colon cancer. It is, as its name suggests, characterized by the appearance of relatively few polyps. In this syndrome, although there are few polyps, a much higher proportion of these develop into malignant cancer. Sufferers from this syndrome have about a 75% chance of developing full-blown colon cancer.

Cancer is so inevitable in people suffering from these two syndromes that a drastic solution presents itself. Since the defective genes result in a predisposition restricted primarily to the colon, removal of the colon has a dramatic effect on the risk. For this reason, patients with such a strong predisposition to colorectal cancer often undergo such surgery. However, because the genes affected in these syndromes are also needed in other tissues, these people also suffer from an increased risk of other cancers.

Inheriting breast cancer

In women, the most prevalent predisposition syndrome is towards the development of breast cancer. As mentioned in chapter 9, a woman's genetic make-up has a strong influence on her chances of developing cancer. However, women who carry a mutation in one of two particular genes (BRCA1 and BRCA2 – BReast CAncer genes 1 and 2), are much more likely to develop breast cancer. When we talk about someone 'having the BRCA gene', we mean the person carries a mutation in one copy of one of these two genes.

About one in eight American women will develop breast cancer. Amongst these women, 5–10% of the cases will be because they have inherited a defective BRCA gene. The chances of developing breast cancer in those who carry a BRCA mutation varies from about 40% to 80%, depending on the precise mutation they carry. In other words, since the risk is most commonly nearer to 80%, if a woman carries the mutant gene, she will probably get breast cancer. Inheriting this strong first step towards breast cancer also leads to an early onset of the disease. About 50% of these women will develop breast cancer before the age of 50. Unfortunately, such women also have an increased chance of developing ovarian and cervical cancer.

The proteins encoded by the BRCA genes are part of the machinery that repairs DNA damage, double-strand breaks in particular. When both copies of one of the BRCA genes in a cell are defective, that cell and its daughters become hypersensitive to DNA damage because breaks are not efficiently repaired. Perhaps the reason that this results in such a high frequency of cancer is that double-strand breaks occur in all cells during their normal replication; they do not require a major carcinogenic event. When BRCA1 or BRCA2 are no longer fully functional, the DNA breaks do not go unrepaired, but attempting repair generates abnormal chromosomal structures and so chromosome instability and further mutations.

Mutations in either the BRCA1 or BRCA2 gene are present in less than 1% of women in the general population (a fact that has been used to argue against general genetic screening). However, even this small percentage leads to a significant contribution to cases of breast cancer. There are over 1,000,000 cases of breast cancer a year worldwide, killing more than 400,000 women annually. These women often develop cancer at a younger age than those who develop other common cancers. Since 5–10% of these cancers and resulting deaths appear to be directly related to carrying a mutant form of BRCA1 or BRCA2, it is not surprising that BRCA has entered our general vocabulary.

Inheriting skin cancer

Another, very rare, example of a cancer predisposition syndrome, Xeroderma Pigmentosa (XP), is worthy of mention. The hallmark feature of this syndrome is increased sensitivity to sunlight. Individuals with XP suffer the usual effects of ultraviolet light but have a much lower threshold of sensitivity. They burn very rapidly and, if exposed at any level, are likely to develop skin cancer, with an average age of onset of eight years. Like the BRCA genes and the genes mutated in hereditary non-polyposis colon cancer syndrome, this disease is a result of defects in a DNA repair pathway. A defect in any one of the genes in this particular pathway leaves a person hypersensitive to sunlight, making them more than 1,000 times more likely to get skin cancer than the rest of us. Why is skin cancer the most notable risk? The particular pathway for DNA repair that is affected is most critical in response to the kind of DNA damage that ultraviolet light induces. Such people are also about 20 times more prone to several other cancers of internal organs, where the same DNA repair pathway exists but is presumably less crucial than in the skin. Unlike those likely to develop colon or breast cancer, sufferers from XP cannot have the susceptible tissue removed to avoid cancer but, since the cancer only occurs with the assistance of ultraviolet light, they can significantly reduce their risk. Children who suffer from this syndrome must avoid sunlight entirely, either by covering themselves in appropriate clothing or only venturing out in the dark.

In familial syndromes such as those discussed above, the outcome for individual members of the family varies. Only some will inherit the defective gene and even among those who inherit a defective gene, the timing and precise type of cancer varies. Why might this be? The answer comes back to the basic mechanism of cancer development. These syndromes are dominant for the risk of cancer but they all require additional mutational events, one of which is usually the loss of their one good copy of the affected gene. These subsequent events are random occurrences, in any cell, in any tissue, at any time. So the actual outcome of when, where and, sometimes, if a cancer forms is down to chance.

Although these syndromes represent only a minority of the world's cancer cases, their study, in particular the discovery of which gene has been damaged, has been an exceptionally powerful route to discovering the pathways that lead to cancer in all of us. The defective genes that are inherited in these cancer predisposition syndromes are often the same genes that must be randomly mutated to give rise to cancers in the general population.

Summary

For most types of cancer a small proportion are not simply sporadic, random events. Instead, they appear because a person has inherited a defect in one of their genes (a tumour suppressor gene) from one of their parents and so every single cell in their body carries that defective gene. As a result, that gene produces a defective protein and just one more mutation in their second copy of that gene in any cell in their body could result in a complete loss of its activity. Most such genes are important to cells of only some tissues and so loss of their function will only matter if it occurs in that organ (P53 is a rare exception to this affecting almost every cell type of the body). Those unfortunate individuals who inherit one of these defective genes do not 'inherit cancer', but they are much more likely to develop cancer since they only require one mutation in one of very many cells of their body for cancer to be initiated.

11

It shouldn't happen to children

Because our cells are normally so well protected from genetic damage, it takes many years for them to sustain enough mutational hits to behave in a cancerous way, so cancer tends to occur in the later decades of our lives. It would therefore seem that cancer should not occur in children, but it does. It may be less common than in adults, but in developed countries cancer is

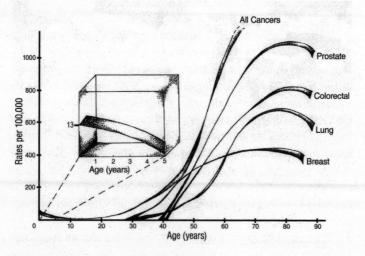

Figure 14 Age distribution of cancers
Insert shows the small peak in childhood cancers in the first few years of life (based on data from 1976 and 1994).

responsible for more deaths in children aged between 1 and 19 than any other disease.

This small peak of cancer incidence in childhood represents a diverse group of tumours of types that appear almost exclusively in children. Rather than their incidence increasing with age, these cancers occur in the young, sometimes the very young, but then their incidence decreases, often disappearing by adulthood. The number of cancers in children is not large; the chances of a cancer arising before 15 years of age is generally less than 1 in 1,000 compared to 1 in 100 in our 50s and 1 in 20 in our 70s. However, cancer is one of the main causes of childhood death, second only to accidents. Strikingly, the most likely time for a child to develop cancer is within their first three years of life, after which their risk declines until they reach adulthood.

Children's leukaemias

The most common of the cancers that occur in young people are leukaemias, cancers of the white blood cells, the main front line of our immune systems. Unlike other types of cancer, in which most mutations result in the loss or changes of individual bases of the DNA, leukaemias more frequently exhibit rearrangements of the chromosomes, in which part of one chromosome becomes fused to part of another. Although carcinogens may play some role in triggering these changes, they are believed to be in part due to a side effect of the way in which our immune system is generated, reflecting its elegant and unique biological mechanisms.

When our bodies are attacked by bacteria, viruses or foreign substances, our immune system recognizes them and produces specifically tailored proteins, *antibodies*, to fight against them. To defend our bodies well, we must generate millions of different antibodies. We would need a huge amount of DNA if each antibody were encoded by a separate gene, but over millions of years a wonderful system has evolved that makes us very good at generating a response to almost any invading agent, using the minimum of our body's resources. Our cells economize by using a relatively small number of genes, which are reorganized into different combinations of their parts to generate many different antibody proteins from each gene. To do this, the DNA is broken and recombined. When this all works accurately, things are fine but occasionally this efficient and remarkably effective strategy for generating diversity backfires and mistakes happen. One type of mistake leads to part of an antibody gene being accidentally joined to another gene on another chromosome, which causes that gene to make too much of its protein. If this other gene is an oncogene, cancer may ensue.

Most leukaemias occur in the elderly but there is an unusually high frequency in the very young, between the ages of two and six. Leukaemias, mostly acute lymphoblastic leukaemia (ALL), account for about a quarter of childhood cancers. The cancer cells of ALL contain the rearrangements of chromosomes typical of leukaemias. Remarkably, as many as one in every hundred healthy newborn babies have been found to have blood cells that already contain a *pre-leukaemic clone* of cells – in which a rearrangement between a gene called TEL and a region called AML1 on another chromosome has occurred. Since ALL only occurs in about 1 in 10,000 children, conversion of these pre-leukaemic cells into cancerous cells is not inevitable. However, the occurrence of this first step towards cancer in the blood cells before birth could provide one explanation why leukaemia occurs in the very young. In babies whose cells have this rearrangement, only one additional mutation needs to occur after birth for these pre-leukaemic cells to have taken two steps towards cancer. And once two steps are taken, the process may be irrevocable and sometimes quite rapid.

Children's solid tumours

While leukaemia represents the most common cancer seen in children, a wide range of solid cancers, appearing in a broad range of tissues and organs, makes up the remaining 75%. The peak incidence for children's cancer is below the age of 10, so it is hard to see how the many rounds of genetic damage seen in the formation of cancers in adults can apply to them. If cancer is driven by mutations and several must occur for a malignant cancer to evolve, how can this be achieved in such a short time?

In all honesty, we don't really know why children get cancer. Three alternative explanations seem possible. Either mutations happen more rapidly in children's cells, fewer mutations are needed to cause cancer or an entirely different mechanism exists. Whichever is true, we must also explain why this rate of cancer development is seen in young children, but the frequency of these cancers decreases rapidly with age.

It is clear that children's tissues are not more prone to cancer than adults' since, despite this small peak in incidence, the numbers of cancers in children are still very low compared to adult cancers. The types of cancer that afflict children are, to a large extent, different from those that affect adults. The commonest cancers of adults, such as colorectal cancer or lung cancer, are very rare in children. The reason for this difference appears to be linked to a general observation: children's cancers arise when the organs involved are growing most quickly. Most types of children's cancer occur in narrow age ranges: some predominate in infants (below the age of three), others in those nearer 10 or 15 years old. There appears to be a simple correlation between the period when the cancers occur and the period when those tissues undergo their highest rates of growth. Since the inheritance of mutations in successive generations of cells requires the cells to be dividing, the association of cancer with proliferating cells is not surprising. The more cells that are dividing, the more opportunity there is for mutations to be acquired.

Is the mechanism underlying children's cancer fundamentally different to adult cancers? I would argue that it is, and that mutagenesis (the induction of mutations by environmental influences) is unlikely to be the driving force. One line of evidence is that, unlike adult cancers, the incidence of most children's cancers shows relatively little geographical variation, despite the known variation in exposure to environmental carcinogens that explains much of the variation in incidence of adult cancers. So why do children get cancer? I believe that it is akin to birth defects. The processes that control our development from fertilized egg to infant are imperfect. This imperfection in the ability of our cells to behave properly as they multiply during embryonic and foetal growth can result in dramatic developmental defects in a significant number of pregnancies. As many as 30–50% of forming embryos are lost before, or at, birth and more than half of these losses are believed to be due to genetic abnormalities. Most are lost during the very earliest stages of the embryo's growth, in the first few weeks of pregnancy. With respect to cancer, and potentially many other abnormalities that occur during embryonic and infant development, errors in DNA replication may be the cause of the problems.

If this DNA damage is not caused by environmental factors, what is its cause? Unfortunately, it seems likely that one of the main causes is simply the inherent imprecision of the DNA replication process. On average, for any given gene, the DNA replication machinery makes a mistake that remains uncorrected and inherited by the next cellular generation, every 10 million cell divisions. In later life, this rate of error is unlikely to cause any problems, since a limited number of cell divisions take place during adulthood. However, during pre-natal and early life, far more cells are dividing as we grow. A major difference between these dividing cells and those in adult tissues is that, to provide the necessary growth in the size of their organs, these cells in foetuses and young children divide again and again and again, providing an opportunity for mutations to accumulate (most dividing cells in adults are destined to stop proliferating after relatively few divisions in order to differentiate into the functional cells of the organ concerned).

A prime example of the association between proliferation and cancer is seen in the cerebellum (the part of the brain at the back of our head), which is responsible for co-ordinating movement and balance. During the first year of life, the cerebellum generates approximately 10 million million million (10^{10}) cells. In that one year, approximately 10 million million million cell divisions must take place, providing ample opportunity for the inherent inaccuracies of the DNA replication machinery to generate a large number of mutations. And so, 1 in 200,000 children under 15 develops a tumour in this region of the brain (a very rare kind of tumour in adults). The same applies to various other organs of the body as they grow, either earlier (the liver, the kidney and the rest of the brain) or later (the bones and the reproductive organs) in life. This does not mean exposure to carcinogens cannot or does not influence the occurrence of children's cancer. Rather, there may be an underlying cause behind many or most of these cancers of childhood, which occurs in the absence of carcinogens and so perhaps cannot be guarded against.

This explanation may also account for another observation in children's cancers. By the time they are diagnosed, most adult cancers have massive damage to the genome, with many fragmented and disorganized chromosomes, due to the genome instability they have developed by this stage in their growth. Although most children's cancers also show genome disorganization, the damage is generally much less than is seen in adults. Indeed, in the cells of a teratocarcinoma, one of the earliest and quickest-developing tumours, most commonly diagnosed in newborn infants, there is often no discernible damage to the chromosomes at all. In adult tissues, the level of cell proliferation is much lower than in developing tissues, so the genome must somehow be destabilized to increase the frequency of mutations, which leads to the massive genome rearrangements. If, at least for some of the mutations that occur in children's tissues, this destabilization is not required, this would explain why the genomes of children's cancers are less disorganized than those of adult cancers. This is consistent with the idea that the mutations in children's cancers are largely due to the high level of proliferation seen in their growing organs.

A second possible explanation for the low level of DNA damage that occurs during formation of children's tumours relates to the tissue environment of the cancer cells. The cells of growing tissues are highly proliferative because the cells around them produce signals instructing them to survive and divide. Therefore, at least in their initial stages, cancer cells in children's growing organs may not need to overcome the need for these signals. Such cancer cells would not need to acquire the mutations, seen in adult cancers, which make them able to grow when growth signals are absent; so children's cells would need fewer mutations to become cancerous.

Treating cancer in children

Children's cancers also differ from those of adults in a way that is probably of more direct concern to most of us. The fact that they are in a developing body has a major impact on therapy. As in adults, the major strategy for the treatment of cancer in children is to target, rather non-specifically, dividing cells. In adults, this can have side effects, such as hair loss and nausea, because the treatment also affects the normal dividing cells of our organs and tissues. In children, especially the very young, many tissues are actively growing and so contain large numbers of dividing cells. A treatment that kills dividing cells can therefore have particularly severe effects in the child's body.

Nowhere is this more problematic than in the brain. Current treatments for brain tumours can kill off large numbers of the cells responsible for producing the growing brain and so brain development can be significantly impeded. This is why brain tumours in infants (below two years of age) are rarely treated with radiotherapy; the balance between effectiveness in killing the cancer cells and damage to the growing brain means that the potential side effects can outweigh any benefits of treatment. Such considerations are the driving force behind research into different ways to attack tumour cells without damaging the nearby healthy normal cells required for the continued development of the child's growing organs.

If the in-built error rate of DNA synthesis plays a significant role in their development, there seems little we can do to avoid cancers in children. We therefore need new treatments that avoid the side effects of radio- and chemotherapy. If, as I have suggested, the cells in children's cancers need to be less abnormal to behave as cancer cells, their behaviour may be more easily corrected. Evidence to support the idea that we may be able to encourage some cancer cells to revert back to non-cancerous behaviour comes from a rare phenomenon, seen almost exclusively in children. A few cancers (for example neuroblastoma, a tumour of the nerve cells), which have the appearance of an aggressive cancer, sometimes spontaneously regress. Neuroblastoma 4s is one of the most aggressive-looking forms of this tumour, with cells spread throughout the body. Despite appearing to be in a very late stage of malignancy, this cancer often suddenly and spontaneously disappears. This suggests that, despite their malignant behaviour, these cancer cells are capable of either differentiating into mature, non-dividing cells or undergoing cell death. The same seems to be true of rare examples of cancers of other tissues. If we can better understand how these cells work, we may be able to design therapies that trigger the cells of other children's cancers to behave like them and trick the cancer cells into removing themselves from the body.

Although we still do not understand how and why children get cancer, the application of modern techniques is expanding our knowledge at an amazing rate. There are significant grounds to be optimistic that new therapies will be developed over the next decade or two, allowing us to move away from the classical treatments of radio- and chemotherapy, which can have particularly severe effects on children's development. However, there is one final barrier, particularly pertinent to cancers in children: each individual cancer is quite rare, so the market for drugs specific to that cancer is equally small. This does not give the large pharmaceutical companies much incentive to pay attention to these cancers. Research into new therapies for children's cancers is almost entirely dependent on the efforts of scientists outside the commercial sector. One hope is that therapies can be developed that will also benefit adults suffering from a more prevalent cancer, which might be taken on by pharmaceutical companies. Otherwise, these drugs can only be developed with financial support from governments and charities.

Summary

Cancer is generally a disease of aging. Although relatively few children develop cancer, it remains surprising that cancer is seen in children at all. Since cancers in children must develop in months or only a few years, and children have less time and opportunity to be exposed to carcinogens than adults, it seems that different mechanisms must underlie childhood cancers. The lower numbers of mutations and other features unique to children's cancers suggest the mechanisms underlying their cause differs from adult cancers, but also provides hope that they may be more responsive to medical interventions.

Part 4
Winning the war

12
Attacking cancer

From the earliest times, it has been recognized that the best way to deal with cancer is to catch it early and hit it hard. Screening programmes have therefore become a significant weapon in the battle against cancer: the earlier a cancer is detected, the more likely it is that treatment will be successful, because the cells have had less time to become abnormal and are less likely to have spread to other organs.

The basic strategies for treatment remain the same today as they have for many decades. Every year, many billions of pounds, dollars and yen are spent, and many millions of hours dedicated by some of the greatest scientific minds in the world to the search for a cure for cancer. Despite this, those of us who are unfortunate enough to find ourselves in hospital suffering from cancer are as likely to be subject to surgery, radiotherapy and/or chemotherapy as we would have been 10, 20 or even 50 years ago.

However, the many decades of intensive study have been far from fruitless: we now know a vast amount about the causes and the biology of cancer. So why has our treatment changed so little? The answer is twofold. First, the basic strategies to kill cancer cells are pretty effective and, despite the apparent lack of change in therapeutic approaches over the years, surgery, radiotherapy and chemotherapy are much safer and more effective than they were even as recently as the 1980s. In particular, rapid improvements in imaging technologies that allow doctors to see tumours in ever-increasing detail mean we can target surgery and radiotherapy much more accurately. Second, in recent years we have begun to witness the appearance of new treatments that have arisen from the research effort; a new era of therapies based on our understanding of the biology of specific cancers is just beginning.

Screening

For a widespread screening programme to be adopted, several criteria must be satisfied. The benefits of screening should outweigh any risk or harm associated with the screening process, the test should be cost-effective and reliable, and there should be the potential for a beneficial change in treatment if the test proves positive. Since most screening methods have significant costs, and some risks, these programmes are targeted at age groups in whom the chance of developing specific cancers is highest. At present, screening is only generally available for cancer of the breast, cervix, bowel and prostate. Each screening programme is very different and varies in the extent to which it is available in different countries.

One of the most important developments in the fight against breast cancer was the introduction of X-ray mammography screening, or mammograms, in the 1970–1980s. This has allowed many tumours to be diagnosed and treated much earlier in their development, catching them before they spread from their original site. Breast cancer screening is believed to save the lives of as many as 1,400 women a year in the UK.

Despite the well-established and widespread implementation of screening for breast cancer, it remains contentious. Many early tumours, which can be identified by screening, do not progress to a life-threatening cancer during the lifetime of the woman in whom they are diagnosed. This is either because they are not very aggressive forms or because the woman will die of something else before the tumour ever became life-threatening. Thus diagnosing and removing the tumour would not have been necessary.

The argument in favour of screening is that such 'unnecessary' surgery is in fact a necessary side effect of ensuring that malignant and life-threatening cancers are found early and removed. Basically, we are currently unable to determine which tumours will be life-threatening and which will not. Estimates of how many women undergo 'unnecessary' surgery vary; the most recent studies indicate that three extra woman undergo such surgery for every one life that is saved. Generally, even those who question the validity of screening programmes do not argue that they should not take place, but rather that women should be better informed of what a positive result means. However, the numbers are often presented in a way that makes such informed consent very difficult. I have therefore included a box here to help you to understand what these numbers would actually mean to you whether you are offered or actually undergo such screening. Despite these concerns, breast-screening programmes remain an important strategy in the fight against breast cancer.

THE STATISTICS OF BREAST CANCER SCREENING

Each time you are screened there is on average a 1 in 90 chance that you will be diagnosed with breast cancer for which surgery and chemotherapy is recommended. This means that if you undergo regular screening as offered by the NHS every 3 years between the ages of 47–73 (8 rounds of screening) your chances of being diagnosed with breast cancer are approximately 1 in 12.

The number of women who are considered to have been 'overdiagnosed' in breast screening has been estimated by comparing how many women are diagnosed with breast cancer in populations of women who have been screened to the number diagnosed in populations that do not take part in a screening programme. This is

THE STATISTICS OF BREAST CANCER
SCREENING (*Cont.*)

an imprecise art and so studies vary in their conclusions. However, the largest and most recent studies are in agreement. Among those who receive treatment just over three out of four women will survive their cancer. However, because of overdiagnosis, it is likely that one in five of surviving women would have survived without any treatment. On the other hand, if the same women had not undergone screening, then approximately one in twelve of the cancers that were survived would not have been detected until it was too late and the therapy would have failed and those women would not have survived their cancer.

This data suggests that if you are screened regularly over a 20-year period, there is, on average, about a 1in 200 chance that this will save your life (i.e. if you choose not to be screened, there is a 1 in 200 chance this decision will be fatal), but there is also, on average, a 3 in 200 chance that regular screening will lead to unnecessary treatment. Both of these risks are likely to go up or down depending on other aspects of lifestyle, such as your weight, number of pregnancies, breast-feeding history, exercise and diet.

If you are diagnosed with breast cancer through screening and you are one of the women who survive after treatment, you will not know if the treatment saved your life or if you are one of the one in five of these women for whom treatment was actually unnecessary. All you will know is that you had breast cancer, you were treated and you have survived.

* The numbers provided are based on the NHS, CRUK and internationally published data at the time of publishing.

Cervical screening is carried out much earlier in women's lives (between 20 and 30 years of age, depending on the country), because the risk of occurrence begins earlier than for breast cancer. The cervical smear test, often called the Pap smear (named after George Papanicolaou, who introduced it in the 1930s), or the more recently introduced liquid-based cytology test, are prime examples of the benefits of screening programmes. This test is designed to detect abnormal cells at an early stage, before they develop into full-blown cancer. The tests work because the normal cells of the cervix are relatively uniform. By analysing cells taken from the surface of the cervix, the presence of any abnormal cells can be determined before they have the opportunity to become cancerous. Even if the test is positive the abnormal cells will often not develop into cancer. However, if the cells appear very abnormal, a biopsy (removal of a small piece of cervical tissue) is usually made, to confirm the result. More recently, the added detection of the human papilloma virus, which causes cervical cancer, has further improved detection rates.

The use of smear tests has dramatically increased survival from cervical cancer. In many developed countries, survival rates are about 70% higher today than they were in the 1980s. However, the picture is not so positive where screening programmes are less well established or where recruitment into the screening programmes is less successful. Unfortunately, although screening is believed to reduce death from the disease by as much as 80%, cervical cancer is often very aggressive. Despite programmes that screen women every one to three years (in many countries), some women are already beyond cure when they are diagnosed. For this reason, this is the first cancer for which, in the West, a vaccination programme has been put in place (see chapter 8, p. 93–94, chapter 13, p. 162).

Until recently, the only cancer in men for which there was a routine screen was cancer of the prostate. This is because it is the most common cancer of men, the test is cheap and relatively non-invasive and the age group at risk is well defined. Prostate cancer is a cancer of the old, so screening begins in most countries from 50 years of age. The most common screens involve a simple rectal examination to feel if the prostate gland appears sensitive or abnormal, and analysis of the man's blood for the presence of high levels of *prostate specific antigen* (PSA – a protein produced by the prostate that is normally only found at low levels in the blood). However, other than in the USA, population-wide screening has not been generally adopted. Even in the USA the United States Preventive Services Task Force has now recommended that healthy men are NOT screened for prostate cancer using these tests. This is due to the analysis of earlier screening programmes in the USA and Europe, which failed to provide convincing evidence that these tests are sufficiently reliable. In particular, blood PSA levels can be high in those without cancer or low in those with cancer. As a result, despite the fact that screening and early diagnosis of this cancer might reduce mortality by 20% (a figure disputed by some studies), it has been estimated that as many as 48 men are treated for every life saved. In other words, mass screening would result in unnecessary surgery (with its associated risks and side effects, such as impotence and incontinence) for many men who have cancerous prostate cells that would never become life-threatening in their lifetime. What is needed is a more reliable test to determine which cancers are more aggressive, and a more conservative treatment option for when it is not certain that a cancer is life-threatening. The latter of these is already more common in many countries so that the screening, even as it now stands, may yet be considered acceptable.

Since about 2002, screening for bowel (colorectal) cancer has begun in several countries. Bowel cancer is a prime target for preventative screening because it is a major killer; in the UK, over 16,000 adults are likely to die from this disease every year. Bowel cancer usually starts as a slow-growing, pre-cancerous polyp, which, if detected, can be removed. Screening generally involves two types of test: the faecal occult blood test (FOBT), which detects small amounts of blood in the faeces not readily seen by the naked eye, and tests such as colonoscopy, which inspect the inner lining of the colon and bowel for polyps. Although colonoscopy is far more sensitive in detecting abnormalities, most screening programmes use FOBT as the more cost-effective method.

Pilot studies suggest that about 2% of people over 50 years of age will have a positive FOBT. Yet follow-up colonoscopy reveals that only one in ten of this group has an actual cancer. The FOBT test means that these cancers are likely to have been detected much sooner than they otherwise would and treatment is therefore likely to be more successful. Another four in ten of those with a positive FOBT will have one or more benign growths or polyps, which can be removed to avoid any risk that they will later transform into full-blown cancer.

However, in addition to about half of the positive results for FOBT turning out to be false positives for cancer, the test also misses a large number of polyps and cancers. Colonoscopy has been shown to detect polyps and cancers in up to four to five times more people than FOBT. So why not adopt colonoscopy as the initial screening method? One reason is cost: a typical FOBT test costs tens of pounds; screening the UK population using FOBT costs about £20–30 million a year. Colonoscopy and similar techniques cost hundreds or even thousands of pounds per test the total cost of such screening would be huge by comparison. Also, the take-up rate of screening using colonoscopy is much lower than FOBT, possibly because some people find it is more uncomfortable and embarrassing. Finally, techniques such as colonoscopy are not without risk: for example, perforation of the bowel occurs in a very small number of cases (fewer than 1 in a 1,000); this might, in exceptional circumstances (about 1 in 10,000 procedures), result in death. In a recent study in North America the death rate from colon cancer in the general population was about 1 in 100, but this was halved in those who underwent screening by colonoscopy. Therefore, for most of us, the benefits of this screening seem to clearly outweigh the risks. Fortunately, in the last few years sigmoidoscopy, a less invasive and cheaper version of examining the rectum and lowest part of the bowel, the sigmoid colon (less than examined in a colonoscopy), has shown great promise. It seems that this will identify many early growths and so reduce bowel cancer deaths significantly (since about 50% of bowel cancers occur in the rectum or sigmoid colon). For this reason, at the time of writing, sigmoidoscopy is being rolled out by the NHS in the UK as a 'one-off' test for those aged 55–60 years of age.

Recent developments in imaging techniques promise a revolution in cancer screening. Colonoscopy and sigmoidoscopy allow doctors to see the actual inner surface of the colon but the use of an invasive camera carries associated risks and unpleasantness. Virtual colonoscopy (CT colonography) uses computerized tomography (also called a CAT scan), in which a series of X-rays is taken and then reconstructed using a computer to provide a 3D image of the colon and rectum. CT colonography is almost as sensitive as standard colonoscopy but costs about a third as much and has fewer of the associated risks, but there is still debate as to whether it should be adopted as one of the main screening methods, due to the risks of repeated exposure to X-ray radiation and relatively poor uptake. It seems likely that this kind of approach, in which internal structures can be examined in ever greater detail, will become cheaper, less invasive and with lower risk over the next few years, so that more effective screening can be developed for a wide range of cancers and for more people. In the meantime, there will still be a great many cancers to treat.

Surgery

The basis of surgery is simple: remove the nasty growth. The reason that other therapies are used alongside surgery is because, unfortunately, it isn't that easy. A malignant cancer is, by definition, capable of spreading. If we simply remove the main tumour, there may already be tumour cells or small secondary tumours elsewhere in the body that will continue to grow and bring us back to the clinic in a worse state than we started. Even if the cancer has not spread, surgery may not rid us of all of the tumour's cells; cells that are left behind or even released from their original site during surgery could grow back or begin spreading, again leading to life-threatening secondary tumours. This is why surgery is normally accompanied either by chemotherapy or radiotherapy, or both, to try and kill any remaining tumour cells and avoid the tumour coming back.

Neither can all tumours be reached by surgery, especially when the tumour tends to grow in amongst the normal cells. If a tumour is in an organ such as the liver or gut, the surgeon may decide that we can do without some of the associated normal tissue and remove the entire tumour and some surrounding tissue, to play safe. However, there are cases, such as brain tumours, where we really don't want to lose even a small amount of normal tissue. Damage to normal tissue is the main side effect of surgery, whether losing pieces of our gut or, after brain surgery, possible disruption of eyesight or muscle control (depending on exactly where the tumour was).

Radiotherapy

The principle behind chemotherapy and radiotherapy is also simple: to kill any cancer cells that remain after surgery. Sometimes, they are also used to shrink the tumour before surgery. Unfortunately, these treatments cannot distinguish which cells are cancer cells and which are not: their aim is to kill any dividing cells. While most features of dividing cells are also shared with non-dividing cells, only dividing cells replicate DNA, so replication of the genome is the focus of most of these treatments. Although they kill off many normal dividing cells, this is generally regarded as a price worth paying, and our bodies can recover from this loss.

The ionising radiation used in radiotherapy, such as X-rays and the radiation from radioisotopes, is the very same type of radiation that can lead to cancer by causing breaks in the DNA strands (chapter 7, p. 83–88). The explanation for this apparent paradox is quite simple. The level of radiation that damages DNA and so causes mutations that might lead to cancer is relatively low. Therapy uses much higher doses of radiation, which the cells should not survive, and so any mutations cannot be carried forward into the next generation of cells.

The levels of radiation experienced when the nuclear reactor in Chernobyl, in Ukraine, exploded in 1986 were enough to cause substantial mutation and damage to DNA, but cells survived and were prone to develop into cancer. Therapeutic doses are beyond those experienced by victims of the Chernobyl disaster. Therapy is a nuclear attack on tumour cells, equivalent to placing them less than two kilometres from the epicentre of the nuclear explosions in Hiroshima or Nagasaki. We want therapeutic radiation to have the same effect as the lethal radiation from an explosion: to damage cells so much that they cannot survive. If this radiation were experienced by our whole body, it would kill us, but therapy targets the tumour as closely as possible. Although healthy tissues can be affected, it is only in a limited area.

Radiation-induced damage can kill cells in several ways. In non-dividing cells, the damage inflicted on their genome causes some to die but most will survive and function. In dividing cells, most cells will initially survive and progress through the cell cycle, despite the many breaks in their DNA. As the cells attempt to divide with a badly broken genome, the genome becomes progressively more damaged until it can no longer go on, and the cells die (a phenomenon known as *mitotic catastrophe*). Massive DNA damage can also trigger P53-driven apoptosis (chapter 3,

p. 37) (if P53 has not been inactivated, as it is in about 50% of cancers). In addition, free radicals generated by radiotherapy can damage other components of the cell, such as cell membrane proteins, which can also trigger apoptosis by other means.

Not surprisingly, such heavy-duty killing of dividing cells is quite effective. However, even when such overwhelming force is used, some cancers contain rare cells that are particularly resilient and survive the treatment, reappearing despite the destruction of most of the tumour. Unfortunately, in many cases we cannot raise the level of radiation high enough to kill off such resistant cells without producing unacceptably severe side effects.

All forms of radiation can damage our DNA. Depending on the exact nature of the tumour, X-rays or radioisotopes are used to generate beams of radiation that can penetrate our body to reach the tumour within. Since this nuclear attack kills normal cells in much the same way as it kills tumour cells, the treatment is limited by the severity of its side effects. This is why radiotherapy treatments are often *fractionated*: the total amount of radioactive treatment is spread out over two, or more, smaller treatments, with a period of recovery in between. Fractionation takes advantage of small differences in the sensitivity to radiation between normal cells and cancer cells, providing time for normal cells to repair the DNA damage and replenish the tissue so it can function.

Another strategy, which is only available in some places but should become more widely available as the machines become smaller and more affordable, is *proton beam therapy*. This makes use of a high energy beam of subatomic particles that can be targeted much more closely to the cancer cells, damaging normal tissues much less than standard radiation using high-energy X-rays and so allowing for more intense radiation of the tumour. This therapy is available in the USA and some European countries, and the first machines able to deliver this therapy in the UK should come on line in 2018. Finally, a technique called *brachytherapy* may sometimes be used, in which radioisotopes are implanted in or near the tumour, so that the tumour cells receive a high dose of radiation with little effect on the surrounding normal tissue. Using these different approaches, radiation therapy remains one of the most effective ways of treating cancer.

Chemotherapy

Although there are many types of chemotherapy agents and many processes essential to cell survival that these agents target, most chemotherapy agents act very much like radiotherapy: they cause alterations to the DNA that interfere with the replication of the genome and so the cells die. Just like radiation, some chemotherapy agents would sit quite happily alongside the carcinogens that cause mutations to occur and increase the chances of a cancer developing. However, just like radiotherapy, the principle of chemotherapy is to drive this process to a point where the cell cannot repair itself and it dies.

The discovery of the usefulness of some chemicals in cancer therapy was the result of an accidental observation. For example, *Nitrogen mustard* was developed as a chemical weapon in World War II; although it was never used, the results of accidental exposure showed it could effectively block the proliferation of white blood cells. Under its chemical name, mechlorethamine, it became widely used as a treatment for lymphocytic tumours (tumours that arise from white blood cells). Mechlorethamine remains in occasional use to this day, but a number of other, similar chemicals have now been developed, primarily to avoid the effects for which nitrogen mustard was originally developed: its ability to severely burn the skin and other tissues.

Although great effort now goes into inventing new chemicals to treat cancer, most of the drugs we use were originally the natural products of bacteria or plants. Mitomycin (which cross-links the two DNA strands in a cell to each other) and bleomycin (which breaks DNA strands) are antibiotics – natural products of one type of bacterium that inhibit the growth of other bacteria. Plants too have found many ways to kill dividing cells, presumably as a defence against parasites and pathogens. For DNA synthesis to occur, the two strands must be unwound and then rewound, otherwise the intertwined strands would rapidly become one enormous knot – this is achieved by the enzyme topoisomerase. Since this process is essential to DNA replication, it has become a target for a class of chemotherapeutics that includes etoposide (isolated from the mayapple plant).

By contrast, vincristine (isolated from the Madagascar periwinkle) doesn't block the replication of the genome, but inhibits its separation into the two new daughter cells. Once copied, the new chromosomes must be pulled apart into each of the new daughter cells. This is the work of microtubules (molecular chains made of many copies of the protein tubulin), attached to two 'pulleys' at either end of the dividing cell. These chains hook on to the chromosomes and drag them in opposite directions. By binding to the tubulin sub-units that make up the links in the microtubule chains, vincristine interferes with the formation of the microtubules and the chromosomes cannot be distributed between the two new daughter cells. Cell division is halted and the cells die.

Side effects

Although they represent our most successful general strategy in the fight against cancer, both radiotherapy and chemotherapy suffer from the same flaw: they target dividing cells – and we have plenty of those in our bodies that we do not want killed. Most of their side effects are due to the unavoidable death of these normal cells.

The degree to which individual organs suffer from side effects usually reflects the degree to which they depend on the production of new cells, as when we lose hair, due to the need for dividing cells in the hair follicles. For both chemotherapy and radiotherapy, the loss of normal dividing cells means that our bodies have to work hard to rebuild that population, and, just like when our immune system is working hard, we feel ill and tired. This is made worse if the blood is affected, sometimes through anaemia (depletion of the red blood cells that carry oxygen around the body).

The chemicals used in chemotherapy are, by nature, toxins. Our bodies are designed to reject such foreign agents and so the chemicals can often make us rather sick. The effects of this are only bearable because we have developed ways to lessen their severity, using other drugs to reduce our body's response, such as agents to reduce nausea and vomiting. The severity of the side effects limits the dose of chemotherapeutic drugs that can be given and so limits their effectiveness in killing the cancer cells. A tumour can only be effectively treated if it is sensitive to a dose of the drug that is significantly lower than the dose that causes unacceptable side effects. One way to overcome this problem is to use *combination chemotherapy*, a combination of drugs that act in different ways. More than 50 different combinations are currently in use, each combination tailor-made to be the most effective against a specific cancer type. Using this approach, the dose of each drug is limited by its particular side effects but the total drug dose to which the cancer is subject is higher and so more effective.

The worst consequences of these therapies are seen in the bone marrow (where new blood cells are produced) and gut. Both these tissues rely on the production of many new cells throughout our life, to replace the many millions of cells they lose every day. The effects on our bone marrow are generally more life-threatening. Some types of mature blood cell (such as red blood cells) can last for as many as 100 days, while others have a lifetime of only a few days. So we need a continuous supply of new cells. All blood cells are produced from a small number of *stem cells* that start life in our bone marrow. These stem cells give rise to rapidly dividing *progenitor cells* from which the mature cell types are finally produced. When the body is subject to chemotherapy, the large numbers of dividing progenitor cells in the bone marrow are hit hard, leading to a rapid decline in the number of mature cells they produce. Because red blood cells are quite long-lived, their numbers don't go down so severely; it is cells with a very short lifespan, such as some white blood cells, that are soon depleted. This leads to one of the most common and acute side effects of chemotherapy, *neutropenia* – the lack of the white blood cells needed to fight off infections. In the worst cases, this can lead to life-threatening infections that must be treated with a combination of antibiotics.

Fortunately, the stem cells from which all other cell types can be produced are relatively resistant to chemotherapy. After a week or two, these cells can replenish all the cells of the blood. But this still leaves the person with a weakened immune system; improving this recovery period is critical. One strategy is to treat the person with *growth factors* that specifically promote the prolif-eration of the cells that repopulate the blood. Unfortunately, in some cases, the effects of the chemotherapy are more severe and affect the stem cell population. This problem can be over-come by bone marrow transplantation; after chemotherapy, the necessary stem cells are put back into the person's bone marrow, and blood cell production restarts. If the cancer being treated is a cancer of the blood (leukaemia), the replacement stem cells must come from another, healthy, person. However, if the cancer is not of the blood and there is little risk that there are any tumour cells in the bone marrow, the stem cells can be taken from the person's own blood or bone marrow (before treatment starts) and replaced once treatment is complete. Bone marrow replacement allows higher doses of chemotherapy to be used, making it more effective against the cancer cells.

In the gut, the side effects of therapy can also be quite severe, but they are generally short-term and the gut tissue recovers well, probably because the cells of the gut are turned over very quickly, so the damaged cells are rapidly replaced by new cells. As in the blood, the new cells are produced from stem cells deep within the gut tissue that are less prone to be damaged by therapy.

The sophistication of the systems for delivering radiotherapy has increased considerably over recent decades. Radiotherapy can be very restricted, targeting just the region of the body where the tumour exists or, at worst, only where tumour cells may have spread. Chemotherapy is usually delivered systemically, to the whole body, via the blood, so the toxic drugs can get equal access to all our body's tissues.

A final problem with both radiotherapy and chemotherapy is that they cause DNA damage, so that cells that do survive treatment might do so with a damaged genome. And so we find ourselves back at the beginning, in a situation that can induce rather than cure cancer. This is why a small number of people develop secondary cancers as a direct consequence of the treatment to cure their existing cancer. The younger the person when they are treated for cancer, the more opportunity there is for the cells damaged by treatment to progress to cancer, increasing their chances of developing cancer later in life by as much as threefold. This is another reason for minimising the number of normal dividing cells exposed to radiation and a driving force in the development of treatments that cannot induce mutations. However, radio- and chemotherapy treatments would continue to be used if their benefits did not outweigh the risk of causing a secondary cancer.

Despite improvements in both radiotherapy and chemotherapy in recent decades, they still have significant side effects, cause considerable damage to healthy cells and are not always successful. Given how much we now know, with the massive advances in DNA analysis since the sequencing of the complete human genome in 2003, we can be reasonably optimistic that a far greater number of new types of therapy, with fewer side effects, will be developed in the next 10 to 20 years, so that the broad brush of radiotherapy and chemotherapy may become the option of last resort for most cancers.

Resistance

It is clear from the many cases where cancers recur after treatment that some cancer cells are resistant to therapy. Resistance often only becomes apparent when a small number of tumour cells reappear after therapy. These cells may be a small, resistant sub-population of the cancer cells that already existed in the tumour; by killing off all the other cells that were not so resistant the treatment promoted the selective survival of these cells. Alternatively, the cancer cells that reappear may have become resistant as a result of mutations caused by the therapy. Although most of the dividing cells of the original cancer would be killed by the treatment, some may have acquired mutations that make them more resistant to the damaging effects of the therapeutic agent. The treatment, by failing to be fully effective and itself creating mutations, causes a new, even stronger, cancer to form.

Summary

Despite the rising rates of some cancers, we are increasingly successful at limiting the number of deaths that these cancers might cause. This is being achieved through several parallel strategies. Screening programmes are extremely important since they provide the opportunity to catch tumours before they become malignant and so give the potential to eradicate the diseased cells, sometimes using less aggressive and damaging treatments. New screening programmes have recently been rolled out and it is likely that more will follow over the next few decades. Surgery, radiotherapy and chemotherapy have now been around for a long time, but they remain the three main approaches applied to deal with cancer when it appears. All three are continuously being developed and altered so even these 'established' approaches are improving year by year. However, the drive for new types of therapy remains strong with many cancers developing resistance to the standard therapies and all of these treatments carrying potentially severe side effects.

13
Prevention and cure: future prospects

Cancer studies, in all their forms, are amongst the best-funded areas of research worldwide and every day sees new discoveries and progress in our understanding. So how are we doing? We have certainly not yet 'cured' cancer. Indeed, until recently we did not seem to be making much headway. When we consider the three other major types of human disease, circulatory, respiratory and infectious diseases, we see dramatic improvements, thanks to our better understanding leading to changes in lifestyle, cleaner environments and improvements in medicine. Only cancer remained relatively constant during the twentieth century.

Since the 1990s, however, the number of deaths from cancer has begun to drop significantly. Research has at last begun to have an impact on many cancers. And because of our interest in cancer, we have learnt a huge amount about how cells and the body normally work. This understanding promises to have even greater impact on our ability to combat cancer over the next 10 to 20 years. Several new treatments are now well established and many more are reaching clinics. The National Cancer Institute in the USA alone sponsors almost 2,000 active clinical trials for cancer treatments. Many of these are testing drugs that target specific signalling pathways necessary for the growth or survival of a particular cancer and these treatments might well lead to alternatives to standard chemo- and radiotherapy.

The problem with the standard treatments of chemo- and radiotherapy is their lack of selectivity. In a sense, these

Rate per 100,000 population

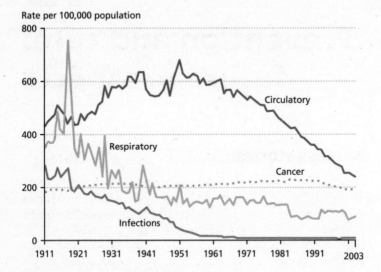

Figure 15 Death rates from different classes of disease during the twentieth century

Source: UK Office of National Statistics.

therapies aim too high, trying to annihilate all cancers. This involves targeting cell division, a feature of cancer cells that is not only common to all cancers, but, importantly, is shared with normal cells. Now, we increasingly think of every type of cancer as an independent disease, able to be targeted by its own therapy.

One of the most common strategies is to find a particular cancer cell's Achilles' heel – an aspect of the cell's biology where it is especially vulnerable but where most normal cells will be immune to the effects of the treatment. Most new therapeutic agents can be divided into two major classes: *monoclonal antibodies* (antibodies produced in the laboratory that possess an exquisite specificity to bind to just one target molecule) and *small molecules* (small chemical compounds that either block or activate specific targets within our cells). Both fulfil a similar purpose; they interfere with very specific molecular targets that have been defined as important to the growth and survival of particular cancers. Many such biological therapies are already in use and more are being tested in clinical trials.

Success stories

Biologically targeted therapies are generally defined as therapies that, by targeting proteins that are naturally present in the tumour cells, either alter a cancer's behaviour directly (for example stopping its growth) or affect the body's response to the cancer cells. Because the pathways affected by these drugs are very specific, they generally only affect the cancer cells and a small sub-population of normal dividing cells, which reduces their side effects.

Given its prevalence, it is not surprising that breast cancer was one of the first cancers to benefit from such new biological therapies. In many breast cancers, hormones (such as oestrogen) are a driving force for proliferation. During the latter part of the twentieth century, this feature of breast cancer cells became a major target for new therapies. Tamoxifen was one of the first (and still widely used) small molecule inhibitors. It works within the breast cells, where it binds with and stops the oestrogen receptor from responding to oestrogen, depriving the cells of the oestrogen-driven growth stimulus. Tamoxifen has had a dramatic effect on the survival of many women; in some studies treatment halved the number who suffered from a recurrence of their cancer.

However, the oestrogen receptor is not present in all breast cancers, and even in those that are sensitive to tamoxifen, the cancer cells can become resistant to this treatment over time. More recently, alternative approaches to target the oestrogen dependence of some breast cancer cells have come into use. In women who have not yet reached the menopause, most oestrogen is produced by the ovaries, so these women are often treated by ovarian suppression, which alters the hormones that regulate ovary function and so inhibits oestrogen production. For women who have passed the menopause, either naturally or if drugs have been used to stop their ovaries working, most oestrogen is generated from the adrenal gland. For these women, aromatase inhibitors can be used to block the production of oestrogen.

A second, well-established, biological therapy applied to breast cancer is the antibody known commercially as herceptin. This antibody binds to a protein, HER2, found on the surface of certain breast cancer cells. By binding to this protein, herceptin causes cell death. Despite being heralded as one of the best new developments in breast cancer treatment, herceptin is only suitable for about one in six women with breast cancer. Fortunately, many new biological therapies for breast cancer are being developed. Some already in use, such as pertuzumab and lapatinib, also target HER2, but in different ways, allowing them to work even against many herceptin-resistant tumours.

Targeting hormone-dependent cancer cells was an approach adopted some time ago in prostate cancer. The hormone testosterone not only plays a key role in the growth of the prostate but also seems to be important in the survival of prostate cancer cells. Blocking testosterone can therefore affect the growth of cancerous prostate cells. The testes are the prime source of testosterone, and in the early twentieth century physical castration was carried out to stop its production. From the 1940s, a better understanding of how our hormonal systems function led to the realization that a similar effect could be achieved chemically. Oestrogen, the female sex hormone, has effects opposing those of testosterone, causing atrophy of the prostate and significantly inhibiting cancer growth. Indeed, *chemical castration*, in which men took oestrogen by mouth, was the first systemic cancer treatment. Oestrogen is no longer widely used, due to its side effects of causing more feminine attributes, such as growth of breast tissue and changes in hair growth, but *androgen ablation* (also known as hormonal deprivation therapy), in which the production and/or the receptors for testosterone are blocked, is much used.

There are biological therapies for a range of other cancers, though most are not yet used routinely. One particular success is the group of drugs that target the activity of a family of enzymes, the *tyrosine kinases*. Tyrosine kinases are a critical part of many growth-stimulating signalling pathways and their activity is often crucial to the proliferation of cancer cells. Whether they are activated by mutations, or simply a normal part of the biology of the type of cell from which the cancer has arisen, the tyrosine kinases are promising targets for new therapeutic agents. Imatinib (also known as glivec or gleevec) is a small molecule that inhibits three of the tyrosine kinases and so can interfere with the growth of tumours where they play a major role. It is now used for the treatment of several types of cancer, in particular certain leukaemias and cancers of the digestive system. Similarly, the tyrosine kinase receptor for the epidermal growth factor is required for the survival of a number of different cancers, so agents that block this receptor can interfere with their growth. These include the small molecule inhibitor, erlotinib, and the antibodies cetuximab and panitumumab, which are already used to treat colon and lung cancers.

Currently, many of the newer biological therapies are used alongside more standard chemotherapy. As more and more such biological reagents are developed, we anticipate that they will be used in combination, overcoming the need to include the more toxic chemotherapies. Already, aromatase inhibitors are being used alongside tamoxifen and various other combinations of drugs in clinical trials.

Another important direction for research into therapeutic drugs is to develop their use as a preventive treatment in healthy people. Breast cancer is likely to be one of the first cancers to benefit from this approach. Researchers have noted that women treated with tamoxifen for a tumour in one breast show a reduced rate of cancer occurrence in the other breast. Although several clinical trials using tamoxifen in healthy women showed a significant reduction in the occurrence of oestrogen-positive breast cancers, the preventive use of tamoxifen has not been widely adopted, as it carries an increased risk of endometrial cancer, stroke, pulmonary embolism and deep-vein thrombosis. Raloxifene, a drug similar to tamoxifen but with less severe side effects, is now approved for use by post-menopausal women at moderate or high risk of developing breast cancer (such as those with a family history) in the UK and US among other countries. Several other agents are now being tested as preventive treatments for a range of cancers.

Many different pathways are being targeted, in many different cancers, and with many different drugs. They provide a number of exciting and promising therapeutic agents, some of which might have a major impact on specific cancers within the next decade.

Targets for therapy

Of course, we want all the treatments we develop to destroy cancer. One of the latest insights in this respect is the identification of *cancer stem cells*, which could explain why some treatments fail to rid us of the cancer. Although many cells in a cancer are still dividing, in recent years it has been shown (albeit in experimental situations) that in many types of cancer only a small sub-set of cancer cells, called cancer stem cells by some researchers, can initiate the formation of a new cancer. Since only these few cells can make a tumour, when cancer recurs after treatment, this group of cells is the likely culprit. The nature and even the existence of cancer stem cells remain contentious, but data suggests that it is less important how many cells of the tumour a treatment destroys than whether it kills the cancer stem cells. Unfortunately, cancer stem cells appear to be rather resistant to standard therapies and much effort is being put into better understanding them, so we can better kill them.

Another way of killing tumours is to starve them to death. Growing tumours depend on blood vessels to provide them with the nutrients and oxygen they need to survive, so anti-angiogenic therapies, which inhibit the growth of these blood vessels, have been developed. Most of these therapies use antibodies that target either the pro-angiogenic protein VEGF (see chapter 4, p. 41), or small molecule inhibitors of the VEGF receptor. This approach is already in use for some cancers of the colon, lung, breast, brain, cervix and liver, and is being tested for many other cancer types. A useful spin-off of this approach is the application of these therapeutic agents to a form of age-related macular degeneration, a disease in which inappropriate blood vessel growth is also a problem. The excessive blood vessel growth within the retina results in a loss of vision in as many as a million people in the USA at any given time. Injection of antibodies against VEGF has proved very effective in halting, and sometimes reversing, the progress of some forms of this disease. This is a dramatic improvement on the relatively limited success, achieved using laser treatment, before this discovery. My mother is one of those who has developed this disease; fortunately, she was diagnosed at a time when this treatment had just become available; it probably saved her sight.

Helping our immune system to attack cancer

As was discussed earlier (chapter 4, p. 49–50), our immune system does appear to be quite good at identifying and killing cancer cells, especially when they enter the blood stream as part of the spreading process. However, cancer cells almost always overcome this by the sheer weight of numbers or by evading the attentions of the cells of the immune system through a process known as 'immunoediting' (chapter 4, p. 51). In addition, cancer cells often have the ability to suppress the immune system through processes referred to as 'immune checkpoints'. In recent years, these mechanisms have become much clearer and researchers and clinicians have developed strategies to overcome them and assist the immune system of the patient in its attempts to kill off the cancer cells. Some of these have shown remarkable success but, like most successful therapies for cancer, they often carry serious side effects. Here I will discuss two rather different approaches. One is to stop the cancer cells from suppressing the immune system and the second is to immunize the patient against their own cancer.

Immune checkpoint blockers

The way that cancer cells suppress the immune system is by exposing proteins in their surface that are a normal part of this system. These proteins are recognized by 'receptors' on the surface of the immune cells and when the two proteins interact the immune cell is switched off. The therapeutic strategy is simple. An antibody that binds to the receptor on the immune system cell is injected and this stops the two proteins from interacting. There are more than a dozen such pairs of proteins and receptors that can switch the immune cells off, but fortunately some play a more major role than others, and these have therefore been targeted. The drugs ipilimumab (Yervoy™) and nivolumab (Opdivo™) are antibodies that bind to two of the receptors, CTLA-4 and PD-1 respectively. These drugs have been used alone or together in trials for a wide range of advanced or recurrent cancers. At the time of writing, particular successes have been achieved in lung cancer and melanoma. Very few current treatments have a substantial impact on lung cancer. It was therefore a significant breakthrough when drugs such as nivolumab were shown to give an average increase in survival of about three months. With respect to melanoma, earlier approaches of using small molecules to inhibit the signalling that drives many of these cancers was shown to be effective initially, but unfortunately, in most cases the tumours returned after only a few months having developed resistance to such drugs. The most recent reports for the new immune checkpoint inhibitors are that one of these drugs alone can result in extension in patient survival to several years and most recently the use of two drugs, ipilimumab and nivolumab, together can result in almost 70% of patients surviving for over two years (54% with no recurrence of the tumours).

There is, however, a major negative consequence of these drugs as they are currently used. Their mechanism is to block the ability of *any* cells to suppress the immune system via PD-1 or CTLA-4. As a result, the immune system can become overactive. This can cause a number of autoimmune side effects in which various organ systems (especially skin, liver and the intestines) can become damaged, even to a life-threatening point. This has led to the therapy being withdrawn for a significant proportion of patients in the trials. For this reason, these drugs are currently only considered for late-stage, life-threatening cancers where other therapies have failed. However, many new drugs targeting immune checkpoints are in development in the hope that some may have less severe side effects, but remain as effective against cancers.

Immunising against cancer

Where an infection plays a role in cancer, vaccination is a very direct means of prevention. It has been very successful against chronic hepatitis B infection in infants in Taiwan, where mass vaccination has dramatically reduced the number of children who develop liver cancer, halving both incidence and mortality between 1981 and 1994.

The most recent example is the development of an effective vaccine against HPV, the virus that appears to underlie almost all cases of cervical cancer. Since 2008, this vaccine has been introduced free of charge in many countries including Italy and Britain for girls aged 12 to 13. Since the vaccine protects against the forms of HPV believed to be responsible for about 70% of cervical cancers, it seems likely that, at an anticipated annual cost in the UK of £100 million, it will save about 400 lives per year. It remains to be seen if such a pragmatic but expensive strategy will be adopted by even more countries to save the lives of more of the 250,000 women who die of cervical cancer every year.

It should eventually be possible to deal with all virally induced cancers in this way, although it may never be economically viable. It has been estimated that vaccination against the main cancer-causing viruses could protect against as many as one in ten cancers in the West. Other than the cancers caused by infectious agents, it is extremely difficult to develop an immunization strategy to prevent cancers appearing, since the cells we want our immune systems to attack are our own. However, clinical trials for several cancers are under way and two major immunization strategies are already in use. Unlike most standard vaccination programmes, they both aim to get the immune system to attack cancers once they have arisen rather than to immunize against cancer arising in the first place. They also rely on the fact that tumours tend to have some proteins on their surface that are either abnormal, or would not normally be exposed to the outside of the cell, and so might be seen as foreign by the immune system. The first approach, like standard immunization, involves injecting the person with a protein, or mixture of proteins, that are present on the tumour. This results in an increase in the person's immune response to these proteins and hopefully an increase in the attack their immune system makes on the tumour. Clinical trials of this approach are still underway, but, so far, the results haven't been very impressive.

The second strategy is a little more sophisticated. For the immune system to mount a successful attack, a specific type of white blood cell, an antigen presenting cell (often one called a dendritic cell), absorbs foreign proteins from the thing the immune system is setting out to attack. The dendritic cell then presents bits of these proteins on its surface to other white blood cells, in a way that activates them to attack any cells on which those proteins are detected. As a therapy for cancer, the dendritic cells are extracted from the patient and either fed with a protein unique to the tumour cells or simply a soup of proteins from the person's tumour. These *primed* dendritic cells are then injected back into the person, so that they can now activate the other cells of the immune system to attack the tumour. Despite some spectacular results in the skin cancer, melanoma, the promise of this approach has yet to be fully realized; nevertheless, it is being developed for use against a range of tumours including prostate, melanoma, colon and certain tumours specific to children with some very encouraging results in terms of quite long-lasting remissions. The only therapy of this kind to be licensed to date for use in the USA in April 2010 – is Provenge for use against prostate cancer.

Pharmacogenomics

Most research now targets individual types of cancer, or even sub-types, such as the oestrogen-positive breast cancers. Most researchers would agree we could go even further, since every tumour is unique, both in terms of the tumour itself and of the person's physiology, as defined by their specific genetic make-up. Perhaps we could tailor individual therapies, person by person.

Such an approach is already on the horizon, making use of our knowledge of the human genome to gain an insight into the very nature of the person and their tumour. Such use of genomic information to help determine the best pharmacological treatment has been termed *pharmacogenomics*. For example, sequencing a person's entire genome might help us identify if they would have an adverse reaction to a drug or if they have a particular version of the genes that metabolize specific drugs, making them more or less susceptible to the drugs' effects. Sequencing the genes of the tumour itself can provide detailed insight into the genetic events that have been disrupted for the tumour to develop. This could help determine which drugs would be most appropriate to destroy that specific tumour.

HUMAN GENOME PROJECTS

For several decades now we have been able to sequence DNA – decipher the precise sequence of bases that make up the code of our genes. In 1990, our ever-increasing technical ability allowed researchers to begin sequencing the entire genome, three billion bases, of one person. At the time this project was started it was a massive undertaking. Large sequencing centres in several countries eventually completed the task in 2003, at a cost of approximately $3 billion and over 10 years of research.

In that time, our ability to sequence DNA improved enormously, becoming both quicker and cheaper. In January 2008, the 1000 Genomes project was launched, in which the genomes of at least 1,000 people were to be fully sequenced, to gain a comprehensive overview of the genetic variations within the human population. It has been estimated that over 200,000 human genomes have now been sequenced worldwide.

These technical advances also led to the possibility of sequencing the genomes of individual cancers. The first completed cancer genome sequences were published in 2009–2010 and have provided huge insights into the types of mutations that occurred in these

HUMAN GENOME PROJECTS (*Cont.*)

cancers. The genome of a skin cancer, melanoma, was found to contain an amazing 33,000 mutations, many of which were of the type induced by ultraviolet radiation, providing further evidence for the role of sunlight in causing this disease. A lung cancer genome had about 23,000 mutations, most of exactly the type we might expect to result from the carcinogens in tobacco smoke, calculated as representing 1 mutation for every 15 cigarettes smoked.

One of the most striking observations in both these examples is the sheer number of mutations, the majority of which do not seem to affect any genes. This provides the first really concrete evidence for the generally accepted model that cancer is a result of a few key genes becoming mutated due to widespread random mutagenesis, with most of the resulting mutations playing no direct role in the cancer process. In 2015 The Cancer Genome Atlas project was completed with the sequencing of 10,000 cancer genomes. This has yielded a massive amount of new insight into the mutations that cause cancer. The benefits of this should become apparent as more drugs are developed that target these newly identified changes that drive tumour development. The UK-based 100,000 genomes project includes sequencing the genomes of tumour cells and healthy cells from about 25,000 patients with cancer with the potential to use this information to inform their treatment.

How feasible is a genomic analysis of individual people and their tumours? Due to improvements in the technology of DNA sequencing, at the time of writing a whole human genome can be sequenced for as little as $2–5,000, depending on the company offering the service. In fact, large sequencing projects now claim to sequence genomes for an average cost of $1,000. It seems likely that, within the next few decades, even a few years, this kind of personalized information could be routinely used in medicine to provide a much more focused and effective route to cancer therapy. Indeed, many cancer trials now include genome sequencing as part of their analysis to understand why tumours become resistant to the drugs being used.

The ability to analyse the entire genome of tumour cells has already begun to provide massive leaps in our insight into tumour biology. By screening the genome of metastatic tumours (those that are known to have spread) and comparing them with the genome of non-metastatic tumours, a *metastasis signature* – the set of genes that marks out a cancer cell as being able to spread – can be determined. In 2005, Massagué and colleagues took this one step further, studying why breast cancer cells metastasized to the bones in some people, but in others metastasized to the lungs. They identified a small number of genes that, when experimentally introduced into breast cancer cells, endowed those cells with the same preference. Such approaches could soon provide new tools to help us predict which tumours will spread and where they might go – tools of immense value for effective targeting of therapies.

New screening strategies

The most attractive goal for any disease is prevention. A key way to achieve this is to detect benign growths before they transform into a more cancerous form. Developments in imaging techniques already suggest they could largely replace more invasive screening techniques such as colonoscopy. Another rapidly developing area is screening of blood and urine samples for minute traces of molecules that indicate the presence of a tumour somewhere in the body. Tumours leak small amounts of their contents into the lymph fluid and blood; these traces can be detected, either to determine the stage of tumour growth or to screen for the reappearance of tumours after therapy. As these tests have improved, it has become clear that the same methods can be used to screen for the initial appearance of a tumour. The potential for such approaches is apparent from the success of the blood test for PSA, the prostate-specific antigen used to detect the presence of prostate cancer.

Attempts are now underway to identify other proteins that can be used as markers for the presence of a range of tumours, such as a study presently taking place in the UK to identify similarly useful markers for breast cancer. In this study, blood from women whose routine mammograms show positive results will undergo *proteomic analysis*, in which the entire complex mixture of proteins in the blood will be analysed to determine if it contains particular proteins only present when a woman has breast cancer. These proteins could provide markers to screen for the presence of breast cancer in the general population, or at least in those at highest risk of developing breast cancer.

It has even been shown that it is possible to detect DNA that has leaked from tumours into the blood or urine. We can analyse whether specific mutated genes are present, indicative of known mutations that mark a particular cancer. This test is currently being developed to screen for the recurrence of cancers with a known mutation, but could also be used in general screening. Promising data has already been obtained for the detection of several cancers, most notably breast, liver and colon cancer, but these tests are by no means routine.

Urine samples provide one of the least invasive methods of cancer screening. To date, urine has been analysed to determine the presence of tumours located in or near the urinary tract, with tests already in use for markers of bladder cancer. Recent evidence suggests that urine may be just as useful as blood for detecting markers of more distant tumours. It seems likely that many more tests will become available that allow us to determine the possible presence of a wide range of cancers simply by analysing blood or urine. The introduction of less invasive screening will mean earlier detection and so more effective treatments.

Cancer prevention

Given how difficult cancer is to treat once it has arisen, it would clearly be preferable to prevent its occurrence in the first place. A large-scale analysis in 2011 estimated that about 43% of cancers in the UK (as many as 50% of cancer deaths) are readily avoidable through simple changes in lifestyle (Table 4). These include not smoking tobacco, avoiding excess exposure to UV light and adopting a more healthy diet and body weight. Indeed, for cancers of the upper respiratory and digestive tracts (lung, larynx, mouth and oesophagus), avoiding tobacco smoke and excess alcohol has been suggested to reduce risk by over 80%. But what can we do in addition to these lifestyle changes to help reduce our risk of cancer even further? There are probably four broad approaches to this: screening, as described previously (this will identify many tumours before they become malignant and so potentially 'prevent' cancer); the development of anti-cancer drugs that can be used prophylactically to prevent rather than to treat cancers; further adaptations to our lifestyles that could be made if we can clearly identify additional agents that promote cancer and those that help to prevent it; and we can develop ways to avoid babies being born with inherited mutations that make them more susceptible to cancer.

Anti-cancer drugs

As has been mentioned above (p. 157–158), some drugs developed for treating cancer could be applied for prevention. In this scenario, the drug would kill cancer cells as they first arise and so stop them from progressing to a truly malignant form. For most anti-cancer drugs this is not yet feasible or desirable, since they come with side effects and a high cost. The only major example in current use is tamoxifen (or raloxifene), which has been

Table 4 Avoidable causes of cancer in the UK

Cause	% of cancers in women	% of cancers in men
Smoking	15.6	23.0
Overweight	6.9	4.1
Alcohol	3.3	4.6
Infections (e.g. HPV)	3.7	2.5
Sunlight	3.6	3.5
Ionizing radiation	2.0	1.7
Lack of fruit and vegetables	3.4	6.1
Other foodstuffs	2.8	5.8
Occupation*	4.9	2.4
Lack of exercise	1.7	0.4
Short /no periods of breastfeeding and use of HRT	2.8	–
Total avoidable cancers	40.1	45.3

Data taken from Parkin, Boyd and Walker BJC 2011 105, S77–S81

* The major risk from occupation is exposure to asbestos but a small occupational effect may be from other factors.

approved in countries including the UK and the US for women with a strong genetic risk of breast cancer.

But are there other drugs that might help to prevent cancer? To date, because most drugs carry significant negative side effects, they would not be considered unless a group of people was at exceptionally high risk of cancer, as in the breast example.

However, one drug has been found to carry significant benefits with relatively mild side effects. That drug is aspirin. Aspirin has been used in one form or another for thousands of years to treat fever, pain and inflammation. It has now been identified as a potential preventative treatment for cancer. In recent decades people who are at a raised risk of cardiovascular disease have often been recommended to take low dose of aspirin daily. Many of these people have now taken aspirin for many years. This has provided a very large group in which to analyse the possible effects of aspirin on cancer. Since aspirin has anti-inflammatory properties and inflammation is known to potentially contribute to cancer development and progression, it was not unreasonable to propose that aspirin could affect cancer risk. Some of the most striking observations were published in 2012, in which the relative risk of dying from cancer were assessed in large groups of people who had taken aspirin over periods of years compared to matched groups who had not taken aspirin. These studies showed that aspirin use led to about a 25–30% decrease in the number of cases of colorectal cancer. In addition, similar but slightly weaker beneficial effects of aspirin have been determined for breast cancer, prostate cancer and several other cancers, and up to 40% reduction in deaths from cancer. The observation that aspirin appears to have a greater effect on cancer deaths than its effect on the occurrence of cancer suggests that it could be affecting cancer progression and spread. Consistent with this idea, analysis of patients in whom cancer was diagnosed revealed that daily use of aspirin was associated with a 25–35% reduction in cancer spread and deaths. It is important to note that all of the above effects are only seen after five years of daily aspirin use.

A problem with these studies is that they show a correlation between taking aspirin and favourable outcomes for cancer. We cannot be 100% certain that the differences seen in people taking aspirin were actually because of the aspirin and not some other aspect of their lifestyle or physiology. They were not 'trials' carried out specifically to answer that question and so have a number of problems that mean we cannot regard them as proof of aspirin's effects. However, given the promising data described above, a large study that aims to recruit about 10,000 people who have been diagnosed with early-stage cancer has been started in the UK. This 'Add-Aspirin' trial is a randomized and controlled study that will assess the effectiveness of adding aspirin to the treatment for several different types of cancer diagnosed at an early stage in their progression (i.e. to see if aspirin stops or delays those cancers returning after treatment). The study will also analyse the side effects of aspirin to determine whether its benefits outweigh its risks.

So, why have we not been told to take a daily low dose of aspirin as a means to reduce the number of cancers and cancer deaths in the UK? The answer is that, like almost all drugs, there are potentially negative side effects associated with aspirin use (primarily bleeding in the digestive tract). Despite this, in 2015, the United States Preventative Services Task Force released a draft statement recommending the use of aspirin for the prevention of colorectal cancer and cardiovascular disease in those aged 50–69. This advice is restricted to those at higher than general risk of cardiovascular disease and not of increased risk of bleeding (such as those with a history of gastric bleeding or with conditions such as peptic ulcers or low platelet count).

Lifestyle changes

Other than the big players like tobacco, UV light and other forms of radiation, identifying factors that could act as carcinogens is rather difficult. Despite this, large studies carried out over long periods of time have managed to identify factors that have weaker effects, such as alcohol and processed red meats. For most other factors there is little evidence of a role in cancer, or the evidence is inconclusive. This has not, however, dissuaded many authors from putting forward unsubstantiated theories on what it is in the modern lifestyle that has led to the high incidence of cancer that we now see. Likewise, many have exhorted the powers of a wide range of foods and supplements that are proposed to have amazing cancer preventative properties; bookshops are full of such unfounded literature. So are any of these assertions likely to be correct?

For some, we have good evidence that they are false. For others, there is some evidence, but it is equivocal, and for others there simply is insufficient evidence, so we cannot rule them out. And, finally, for a few there is now good evidence that they do play a role in cancer risk. I will pick some key examples of each.

Food

It is not unreasonable to suppose that aspects of our daily diet might protect us from cancer. Our regular food intake represents a daily dose of many different vitamins, minerals, proteins, etc. So, if some of these help the processes that could protect our cells from cancer, then we could be getting them on a very regular basis. Indeed, just as some parts of our diets have been identified as 'bad' with respect to cancer risk, others have been found to be good, such as fibre, fruit and vegetables. However, the effects of these dietary components on risk of developing most cancers is relatively small. A healthy diet high in the good foods and low in the bad will significantly reduce your risk of cancer (perhaps helping to avoid 1 in 10 cancers), but there is no diet that will effectively protect you from most cancer risk.

Green tea

Teas, in particular green teas, have received significant attention due to the particular chemicals they contain (in particular cate-chins) and the association of low risks of certain cancers in coun-tries where people drink large quantities of green tea. Although there have been many studies to look at the effect of drinking green tea on cancer risk, the results are mixed and overall incon-clusive. It seems possible that green tea is protective, but if this is the case it may be restricted to those who regularly drink many cups a day, as is more typical in Asia. It also remains possible that the lower cancer risk in many Asian countries is linked to other lifestyle factors that go alongside drinking green tea.

Exercise

Large studies such as those that identified alcohol and red meats as contributing factors to cancer were also able to assess the link between levels of exercise and cancer. These studies found that the more exercise a person does the less likely they are to develop cancer, regardless of other factors such as body weight (although obesity is also clearly associated with increased cancer risk). In other words, for people of a given BMI on similar diets, those who lead a more sedentary lifestyle are more at risk of developing cancer than those who exercise. Indeed, the more exercise you do, the stronger the protective effect.

Herbicides and pesticides

It has long been known that many chemicals used as herbicides or pesticides in the agricultural industry are mutagenic and sometimes carcinogenic when tested on cells or in animals. However, the doses required to have such effects are typically much greater than the amounts found in the food we eventually buy. For this reason, the chemicals are still in use and we routinely ingest them in our diets. However, it has been pointed out that we eat small amounts of each chemical, not just one, so the intake of potentially toxic chemicals is the total of adding all of these together. The effect of such complex mixtures of chemicals has not been thoroughly analysed. Likewise, we eat these foods regularly over very long periods of time, and this again is hard to mimic in the lab, where animals such as mice only live for a few years. Hence, it would be wrong to say that we know that these contaminants in our food do not play a role in promoting cancer. However, those people who eat more fruit and vegetables have been found to have a slightly lower risk of cancer, so it seem unlikely that the amounts of these chemicals that are ingested with fruit and vegetables can override the positive effects of the foods themselves. It should be noted that people who work with pesticides, and so are regularly exposed to higher doses, may have an increased risk of cancer, but again the evidence is weak.

Mobile phones and electricity power cables

Devices such as mobile phones emit low levels of radiation known as 'non-ionizing' radiation. As the name suggests, this means that unlike powerful, ionizing radiation (chapter 7) this radiation is a much lower energy form that is insufficient to alter the structure of chemical elements. We may be exposed to several types of non-ionizing radiation such as radiowaves, microwaves and electromagnetic fields. Because of the known ability of radiation to cause damage to DNA and so potentially cause cancer-promoting mutations, devices such as mobile phones and exposure to the radiation around electrical power lines and radio masts have been proposed as possible causes of cancer. So do these pose a real risk of cancer? The short answer is that the evidence to date suggests they do not. The level of radiation associated with these devices has been shown to be insufficient to damage DNA (the energy one would be exposed to from phone masts and radio masts is even lower than from the mobile phones themselves). Despite some early small studies suggesting that there could be a link between mobile phone use and the risk of certain brain tumours, much larger and more robust studies following hundreds of thousands of individuals found no such link.

As for high-power electricity cables, which generate electromagnetic fields, the evidence is less clear. It has been reported that numbers of childhood leukaemias are higher in areas where exposure is greatest but it has proven very difficult to carry out studies that clearly test this possibility. The major organizations that monitor cancers have therefore stated that an effect cannot be ruled out, but that any increased risk would only be for those exposed to the highest levels and the effect would be small. It also remains unclear by what mechanism the electromagnetic fields would have such an effect.

Many aspects of our lifestyles have been proposed to increase or decrease our risk of cancer with poor or no evidence to support these claims. These include eating processed sugars, artificial sweeteners, acidic diets and having a positive attitude. I do not have space to discuss all of these in detail here. I recommend visiting the American-based National Cancer Institute or Cancer Research UK's websites where the evidence regarding these is discussed at more length.*

Most of the above advice about diet and lifestyle also applies to those already diagnosed with cancer. In general, a healthy diet will help recovery and may have a small effect on the chances of recurrence, although there is no robust data to support or refute this. There are many, many books on diet for those who have cancer and to supposedly prevent cancer. In general, they promote the healthy diets discussed, but most overstate the case that it will make a big difference. One that I can recommend is *The Royal Marsden Cancer Cookbook*, edited by Clare Shaw. This book recognizes that there is no 'special diet' for people with cancer, but rather provides many recipes based on the available evidence of what makes a healthy diet, with a particular focus on some of the difficulties that come alongside cancer treatments such as nausea, taste changes and sore mouths.

* For more on this, you can go to www.cancer.gov/about-cancer/causes-prevention/risk/myths, www.cancerresearchuk.org/about-cancer/causes-of-cancer/cancer-controversiesorscienceblog.cancerresearchuk.org/2014/03/24/dont-believe-the-hype-10-persistent-cancer-myths-debunked/

TEN RULES TO REDUCE CANCER RISK

The major organizations that fund and monitor cancer research are in clear agreement on the lifestyle changes most likely to reduce the risk of cancer occurring in people who live in developed Western countries. If you have read all of the chapters of this book to this point, you will already know them:

1. Avoid the known major carcinogens: tobacco, asbestos, sunlight/UV light.
2. Limit intake of foodstuffs known to contribute to cancer: red meat, processed meat, meat cooked at high temperatures, salt.
3. Don't drink excessive amounts of alcohol (i.e. more than the health experts recommend).
4. Increase intake of 'good' foods: fruit, vegetables, pulses, etc.
5. Avoid becoming overweight.
6. Do plenty of exercise.
7. Check regularly for lumps or abnormal growths and check with your doctor if you find anything.
8. Breastfeed babies for longer.
9. Only use HRT where absolutely necessary (i.e. when the benefits to you outweigh the increased risk of cancer).
10. Get immunized against the Human Papilloma Virus (now routine for girls in school in most developed countries) and practise safe sex.

Following all of these guidelines will dramatically reduce your chances of developing cancer. And you already know that pretty much all of these rules represent what we might generally call a 'healthy lifestyle'. This means that following the rules will also make you feel better, give you more energy and protect you from many other illnesses and diseases, most notably heart disease and diabetes.

Cancer-free babies

A final strategy for avoiding cancer again reflects our understanding of the human genome. We are all more or less prone
to develop specific cancers: for example, inheriting a mutant
version of a BRCA gene makes us much more susceptible to
breast cancer. For many years we have been able to screen for
such mutations in adults, foetuses and even embryos (conceived
through *in vitro* fertilization, literally meaning 'in glass', that is,
outside the womb), making it feasible to avoid the birth of babies
with the mutation. In other words, if the BRCA mutation is
known to be present in a family, screening can be used to avoid
the birth of children with that mutation.

Screening embryos before they are implanted into the mother
is called Preimplantation Genetic Diagnosis (PGD). When
embryos are created outside the womb, single cells can be taken
from the early embryos and genetically screened (the remaining
cells are perfectly capable of developing into an entire embryo).
Only embryos that have not inherited the defective gene are then
implanted into the mother's womb. This type of test was first
used for the severe inherited cancer predisposition, Li–Fraumeni
syndrome; in 2001, a child was born in the USA who had been
screened as being free of the mutant gene carried by its parents.
In 2006, the regulatory body in the UK added cancer predisposition to those conditions for which pre-implantation genetic
diagnosis is permissible; the first baby to be screened in this way
was born on 9 January 2009, selected because she had not inherited the mutant BRCA gene from her parents. Since then the list
of genes and cancer related disorders for which this procedure
is licensed has grown dramatically to include most major cancer
predisposition syndromes.

The ethics of designer babies is, naturally, the subject of great
debate, but we will certainly be ever more capable of screening for various levels of predisposition to cancer and ever more

interventions will be possible. Whether they are desirable is something for us all to decide.

The future

It is safe to say that we are in a new age of understanding of cancer and genetics that will revolutionize the way we approach this disease. It is also clear that we have entered a period in which progress in diagnosis, treatment and even prevention of cancer is happening more quickly than ever. Between 1970 and 2011 (the most recent statistics available), survival from many cancers has improved dramatically, with average survival from all types of cancer increasing from about 25% to 50%. Even since the start of the 21st century, substantial improvements have been seen for some cancers such as myeloma (improving from about 14.5% to 32.5% 10-year survival) and prostate cancer (improving from about 62% to 84% 10-year survival). Although we cannot yet say that we have cancer on the run, it seems that such a positive view may soon be justified. Many of these advances may come too late for most of us, but they certainly provide real hope for our children and grandchildren.

The sequencing of the human genome has had, and will continue to have, a particularly significant impact on our ability to understand cancer. It seems highly probable that sequencing the genomes of people and their cancers will provide the level of understanding we really need to design new therapies and to tailor those therapies to every person who is unlucky enough to suffer from cancer.

And what can we personally do to help in the fight against cancer? Wherever possible, we should avoid manufacturing, selling or exposing ourselves to any of the cancer-causing agents I have discussed. If we all did that, cancer would be a much less common problem, and our efforts could be focused on solving those cancers that are truly unavoidable.

Summary

It is only in the last 25 years that approaches differing from standard surgery or chemotherapy have become available to combat cancer. Given the rapid advances being made in understanding and analysing genomes and the speed at which new drugs can now be developed, ever more specialized treatments seem likely. Combining new approaches in screening, drug target identification and drug development seems certain to continue the improvements in cancer survival rates over the coming decades. One optimistic view is that within another 25 years cancer will cease to be predominantly fatal, but will be regarded as a chronic disease, most often managed by drugs, as has become the case with diseases such as HIV or diabetes.

Appendix 1
DNA replication and the cell cycle

For a cell to divide, its DNA must be duplicated, the sequence of bases being perfectly replicated. This is achieved by separating the two original strands of DNA from which each chromosome is made and copying a new partner strand for each one. To each base, a complementary base is added, the A base always complementary to the T base and G complementary to C. If we were able to magnify the cell to a point where we could see this happening, the DNA would look like a huge beaded necklace, made up of two intertwined strands of four different types of bead, with a bunch of machines (called *polymerases*) running along its length, building a copy necklace with the same order of beads for each strand. Each of those machines would be selecting the necessary bead from the soup in which this process was taking place and adding 50 new beads to the necklace every second. Despite the many millions of chemical sub-units (about 250 million in humans) that must be linked together in a precise copy of the original genome, our cells can do this in only a few hours. Even at this incredible speed of synthesis, if there were only one polymerase, it would take months to copy the DNA in one cell, so many machines work at different points on the chain to complete the process.

The cell cycle, the series of processes by which a single cell grows and divides to produce two new daughter cells, has four phases. The first is G1, a gap (or growth) phase, in which the cell goes about its ordinary business of staying alive, generating energy

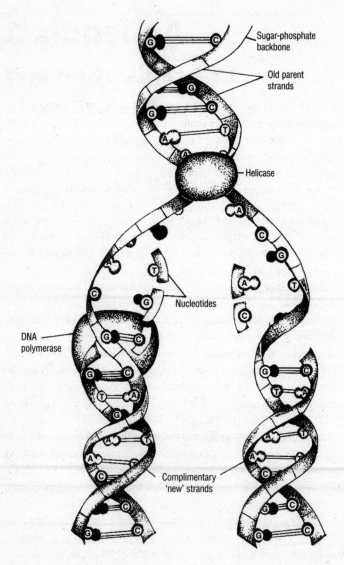

Figure 16 DNA replication

from sugars and making proteins and other cellular components. If it is destined to divide, it will begin to generate more of its cell contents, but only when it enters the next phase, S phase, does it begin to replicate its DNA. In S phase, new strands of DNA are synthesized using the existing DNA of the cell as a template. This is followed by another gap phase, G2, in which the cell continues to grow and make proteins. Finally, there is the rapid M phase, lasting only about one hour, in which the paired, identical chromosomes are pulled apart from each other. Critically, one copy must go to each end of the cell before the cell divides. This is achieved through the assembly of a *spindle*, made up of large filaments, *microtubules*, which extend from *centrosomes*, structures found at either end of the cell. The filaments form a basket-like framework, at the centre of which the chromosomes are attached.

When all the chromosomes are attached to the filaments, one copy of each chromosome is dragged toward either end of the cell as the filaments contract back towards the centrosomes. Once the chromosomes have been separated into the two halves of the cell, a nuclear membrane grows around them, to provide a new nucleus for each daughter cell. Then the cell divides, in the process of *cytokinesis*, in which a number of filament proteins form a draw-string around the middle of the cell which then contracts, creating a deep furrow. As this is happening, more membrane is synthesized to divide the two new cells, eventually cleaving them when division is complete.

The complex events of DNA replication and chromosome separation must be synchronized with cytokinesis, the actual splitting of the cell into two. Not only must the final division of the cell happen only after the chromosomes have separated, but it must happen in a plane perpendicular to the orientation of the separation of the chromosomes, leaving one set of chromosomes in each daughter cell. There appear to be many potential mechanisms that achieve this link between the two processes and it is not yet clear if all cells use precisely the same means.

However, two main strategies have become apparent. The physical events of furrow formation and contraction in the centre of the cell are in some way triggered by the spindle structure that pulls the newly replicated chromosomes to other end of the cell. Thus, the furrow forms at a position equidistant between the two centrosomes. This kind of mechanism ensures both the position and timing of cell division are correct. In addition, the signals that drive the other aspects of the cell cycle are also needed to initiate cytokinesis.

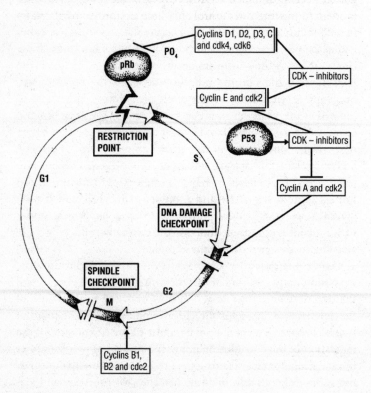

Figure 17 Regulation of the cell cycle

Each phase of the cell cycle is tightly controlled and organized to ensure that all steps are complete and co-ordinated. In general, the cycle is run by a series of proteins that themselves cycle, their levels in the cell increasing and decreasing as the steps of the cell cycle progress. These proteins are, aptly, called the *cyclins*.

Entry to the next round of DNA synthesis in S-phase is regulated at the restriction point by the tumour suppressor protein, Rb. Similarly, P53 is the key arbitrator of whether the cycle can pass the DNA damage checkpoints. Both Rb and P53 interact with the cyclins and their CDK (cyclin-dependent kinases) partner proteins to mediate this control and these are further regulated by the CDK-inhibitors. The Rb protein is controlled by phosphorylation (PO_4) triggered by cyclin/CDKs – when Rb is phosphorylated, the cell cycle can continue. The spindle checkpoint is the final stage when the cycle can be arrested if all necessary events are not complete for mitosis to take place successfully.

As a new daughter cell is born it enters the G1 phase and the synthesis of a cyclin begins. Its level increases to a point where it is sufficient to help the cell enter the next phase, S, when DNA synthesis takes place. As the cell progresses through the cell cycle, different cyclins regulate each phase. The cyclins do not act alone but bind to, and activate, partner proteins, CDKs. These enzymes can add a phosphate to other proteins, so activating or inhibiting their functions. The cyclins and CDKs are actually families of proteins; there are more than eight CDKs and at least four cyclins.

Numerous inhibitors of the cyclin/CDK complexes can jam the cycle at almost any stage. These CDK-inhibitors moderate the activity of the cyclin/CDKs; as part of a system of failsafe switches they represent a series of controls or checkpoints, where the process can be paused or stopped if things are not right. For example, the switches can be tripped by DNA damage, so that a cell cannot continue to divide if its DNA is imperfect, avoiding the passing on of damaged DNA to new daughter cells. Finally, only when specific cyclin/CDK complexes are inactivated can cytokinesis take place.

Controls and checkpoints

The controls that determine whether the cell cycle progresses can be divided into two types. First, the single restriction point stands alone as the key sensor for outside signals that influence whether the next cycle of DNA synthesis is initiated. Second, other checkpoints look inwards to determine if the steps in the cycle are complete and accurate.

The restriction point comes towards the end of G1, shortly before the cell enters S phase and begins DNA synthesis. At this point, the cell assesses whether signals from other cells of the body are instructing it to divide. The decision is controlled by the retinoblastoma protein (Rb). Rb acts like a clutch: unless it receives specific signals, it dislocates key drive proteins from the cycle. Only when growth signals activate the expression of specific cyclins can they activate their associated CDKs, which then turn Rb off (by adding phosphate groups to the Rb protein) and so the cycle can progress to DNA synthesis in S phase. The cell then continues through the cell cycle, all the way back to the restriction point, independent of outside influence. This is therefore a critical point, committing the cell to divide. Since the central event in this signalling process is the inactivation of Rb, which would otherwise stop the cell from entering the next round of cell division, Rb is one of the most important proteins that must be disrupted for a cancer to form. If Rb does not function correctly there is no need for the outside influences to tell the cell to divide – the cell is growth-factor independent.

The second set of checkpoints assesses events inside the cell. These are the DNA replication checkpoint, the DNA damage checkpoints (which exist at several points in the cell cycle) and the spindle checkpoint, which acts during M phase. The DNA replication checkpoint ensures that replication of the genome is complete before the cell cycle continues. If DNA replication is not complete by the time the cell is ready to enter the next phase of the cell cycle, this is sensed and a signalling pathway activated that blocks the cyclin/CDK complexes and halts the cell cycle until the problem is fixed.

There are several DNA damage checkpoints, policed by 'gatekeeper' proteins that check for DNA damage and halt the cycle until repair is complete. Most important among these gate-keepers is the P53 protein, which acts by blocking cyclin/CDK activity. Like Rb, the central role of the P53 protein in this key quality-control process explains why mutations in P53 are seen in a huge proportion of cancers, regardless of their type. In effect, P53 is the key regulator that protects our cells from dividing when the DNA has been damaged by carcinogens. The check-point machinery switches the cycle off to allow the massed forces of DNA repair to do their work.

The spindle checkpoint blocks the cell cycle if the machinery that separates the newly formed chromosomes is not ready. It currently seems that two proteins, Mad and Bub, are key to this. When chromosomes are not already tethered by a spindle, Mad and Bub can bind to the chromosomes. This causes these proteins to signal a stop in the process of pulling the chromosomes apart into the two future daughter cells. Only when all chromosomes are attached are no chromosomes free to bind to Mad and Bub, so this block to the process is removed. Errors at this stage of the cycle are devastating, since the chromosomes will be pulled apart when some are not yet attached, resulting in the wrong number of chromosomes in the two daughter cells.

Recent studies suggest almost 500 genes make proteins directly involved in the cell cycle. However, the key proteins that control entry into the cell cycle and the protection against cell division when DNA is damaged, Rb and P53, are the final arbitrators of the processes. Although each has closely related siblings (P103 and P107 for Rb and P63 and P73 for P53), Rb and P53 (and the pathways in which they function) are most commonly affected in cancers and appear to play the most critical role in cell cycle regulation.

RAS and MYC

For each signalling protein, a different signalling cascade communicates messages to the cell nucleus. The components of these cascades can often be activated by individual point mutations that have a dramatic activating effect on the protein. One of the most commonly mutated genes of this type in cancers is the gene that produces the protein RAS. Many growth factors bind to the tyrosine kinase receptors and many work by activating a RAS protein. The activated RAS proteins do lots of different things, affecting cell proliferation, cell growth and cell survival. Given their central role in mediating growth signals and the wide-ranging effects they elicit, it is not surprising that RAS proteins are often found to be mutated in cancer in such a way that they are always active and so promote abnormal growth features.

One of the key targets of RAS signalling, and indeed many growth signals, is the protein C-MYC. C-MYC is one of the cell's many transcription factors (proteins that directly switch other genes on and off). There are hundreds of transcription factors, many of which activate the cell cycle, but C-MYC is one of the most commonly affected genes of this type in cancer. It is implicated in a wide range of cancer types, including solid tumours of the gut, breast and brain, as well as some leukaemias. Although this gene can be activated by mutations that alter the protein it encodes, it can also play a role in cancer simply as a result of an increase in the amount of the C-MYC protein produced.

One way this is achieved in cancers is by gene amplification. In this situation, the region of the chromosome that includes the C-MYC gene (or its close relative N-MYC) is replicated many times, creating many copies of MYC and nearby genes. Sometimes this forms a separate mini-chromosome, made up only of these repeated sequences. We have little idea of the mechanism behind gene amplification or the reason why it is associated particularly with this gene and with specific cancers. However, no matter what mechanism causes increased levels of the MYC proteins, their over-expression is a very common feature in human cancers.

Appendix 2
How DNA is repaired

DNA is protected from the damaging consequences of carcin-ogens by a broad range of defensive mechanisms. The most common form of DNA damage caused by carcinogens is in the form of chemical alterations to the bases of DNA: base adducts. The simplest way for the cell to correct such structures is by removing the adduct group. In some cases, the abnormal base may be immediately recognized and the chemical alteration reversed. In other cases, the modified base will be removed and replaced (by the base excision repair machinery) or the entire nucleotide may be removed (by the nucleotide excision repair machinery).

If a lesion is not removed, it is likely that the altered base will be misread during DNA replication and the wrong base inserted in the new DNA strand, creating a mutation. Two possibilities for avoiding the occurrence of such mutations now come into play. One solution uses a special form of the enzyme, DNA polymerase, which synthesizes the new DNA strand, to copy the abnormal bases. This special form of DNA polymerase places the correct bases into the new strand, thus making a good copy of the DNA across the lesion (trans-lesion synthe-sis). However, if the adduct is not removed, and an incorrect base is inserted into the DNA when it is replicated, a mismatch is formed in which the added base in the newly forming DNA strand does not pair correctly with the original base on the template strand.

When the polymerase that has just made the new strand of DNA creates a mismatch, two lines of defence are activated. First, the enzyme might immediately recognize the mismatch and back-track, eating away the newly formed strand and trying again (proof-reading). Second, the mismatch may be recognized by the mismatch repair (MMR) machinery. The MMR machinery breaks the DNA, removes the incorrect base and a polymerase and resynthesizes the DNA.

Appendix 3
How infectious agents cause cancer

Epstein-Barr virus

Epstein–Barr virus infection causes proliferation of lymphocytes in about half of infected teenagers, leading to the disease known as infectious mononucleosis. The virus appears to achieve this through the direct action of the proteins it encodes. In Burkitt's lymphoma and nasopharyngeal cancer, the mechanism is not certain, but one viral protein in particular, LMP1, is a strong candidate. When over-expressed in B-lymphocytes this protein increases their proliferation and protects them from apoptosis. Also, its experimental over-expression in mice results in the formation of lymphomas.

Hepatitis virus

Infection with a hepatitis virus carries a risk of initiating cancer of the liver. It is not entirely clear how this virus contributes to liver cancer. The mechanism is likely to involve several aspects of the virus's lifestyle, since some viral genes can promote proliferation or inhibit DNA repair, while the virus genome might sometimes enter the cell nucleus and disrupt important genes, which could also affect key aspects of the cell's biology.

However, it seems that a major contribution to cancer is the inflammation that results from infection. This causes degeneration and consequent regeneration of liver tissue. The increase in proliferation and a local increase in signals from cell to cell instructing other cells to proliferate and to avoid cell death are known to facilitate further mutational events.

Human Papilloma Virus

Most cases of cervical cancer are associated with infection by a Human Papilloma Virus (HPV). This virus has a direct effect on the proliferation of infected cells, because it contains genes classed as oncogenes. These genes, E6 and E7, disrupt the P53 and Rb proteins, central to regulating cell proliferation and survival. The result is that infected cells can proliferate even when signals outside the cell do not encourage them to do so and even when their DNA is damaged. Hence, they over-proliferate and accumulate mutations, a combination that is a powerful driving force for cancer.

Human Immunodeficiency Virus

Human Immunodeficiency Virus (HIV) causes a gradual loss of a crucial type of cell within the immune system, the T-lymphocyte. An increased risk of cancer is just one of the consequences of this immune deficiency. When the immune system is decimated by HIV infection, the body is left susceptible to the rampant proliferation of any potential cancers. In fact, because the body is less able to fight off infections, cancers induced by other viruses are highly prevalent amongst AIDS sufferers. The AIDS epidemic was marked by the rise in a hitherto rare cancer, Kaposi's sarcoma, a cancer of the skin's blood vessels triggered by infection with a herpes virus. Patients suffering from AIDS are also more prone to develop cervical cancer (associated with HPV) and lymphoma (associated with Epstein–Barr virus), although the ability of the HIV to alter directly the biology of the B-lymphocytes through which these tumours arise may also play a role.

Appendix 4

Inherited predispositions to cancer

Li-Fraumeni syndrome

This syndrome is very rare, occurring in only a few hundred families worldwide. However, like many such syndromes, study of these families has been of exceptional value to understanding of cancer.

Sufferers carry a very high risk of a wide range of cancers, most commonly leukaemia, breast, lung and/or pancreas cancer and the brain tumour glioblastoma. Because those suffering from Li-Fraumeni syndrome are born with an initial mutation – a defective copy of the P53 gene – these cancers often arise during childhood. The protein encoded by this gene plays a crucial role in interrupting the cell cycle when the DNA has not been correctly replicated and, when DNA damage is severe, assisting in the decision for the cell to die. A cell that carries one defective copy of the P53 gene only becomes cancerous when the good copy of the P53 gene is also damaged, but any cell in which the second copy of P53 becomes defective will almost certainly form a cancer. The reason why Li-Fraumeni syndrome includes a general predisposition to cancer is the key role of P53 in protecting our genomes from damage in all cell types. By the same token, this is why P53 is so often damaged in sporadic cancers.

Familial adenomatous polyposis

The gene affected in this syndrome was identified in 1991 and named APC after the symptoms (adenomatous polyposis coli – multiple benign tumours of the colon). Individuals who suffer from this syndrome carry one defective copy of the APC gene. The initiation of cancer (that is, the formation of polyps) requires disruption of the remaining good copy of the APC gene. This second event is quite common, as shown by the development of many hundreds or thousands of polyps in those with the defective gene.

This high frequency of loss of the good copy of the APC gene is in part due to the phenomenon of *loss of heterozygosity*, in which the good copy of the gene becomes replaced by a copy of the defective version. Since this is less random than a new mutation appearing in the good copy of the gene, it occurs at a much higher frequency and explains why so many polyps appear in these individuals. Once a polyp is growing, it has a much higher chance of transforming to full-blown cancer because more proliferation results in more mutations. Inactivation of APC has also been suggested to directly cause some destabilization of the genome. Therefore, the more polyps that form, the greater the chance of cancer developing.

The association of mutated APC with cancers of the colon appears to reflect its particular role there. As a result of its key role in cell division, disruption of both of the cell's copies of this gene results in hyper-proliferation and the formation of a polyp. However, APC is part of a signalling pathway, the Wnt pathway, which plays many different roles in many different organs. Therefore, the inherited defect in APC also sometimes leads to the formation of tumours in other organs. The original family in which this syndrome was identified by Eldon J. Gardner developed a range of other lesions, most prominent of which were benign bone tumours (especially of the jaw) and sebaceous cysts (small tumours of the skin). It seems that the specific mutation within the APC gene determines whether it will lead only to colorectal cancer or is likely to also give rise to these other growths, illustrating the complexity of the mechanism by which this large protein works.

Another, independent, syndrome is also due to mutation of the APC gene. Turcot syndrome also exhibits a very high frequency of polyps and colorectal cancer. However, these sufferers also frequently develop a malignant brain tumour, medulloblastoma. Again, the specific mutation seems to explain the difference between the clinical features of Turcot syndrome and those of familial adenomatous polyposis. Since its discovery in these rare disorders, it has become clear that APC is also very commonly mutated in sporadic colon cancers.

Hereditary non-polyposis colon cancer

Hereditary non-polyposis colon cancer (HNPCC) is the second major syndrome in which the colon is the predominant site of cancer. It is characterized by the appearance of relatively few polyps. Like familial adenomatous polyposis, HNPCC is inherited as a dominant predisposition to develop cancer. However, unlike familial adenomatous polyposis, when the second, good copy of the gene is lost, this does not automatically generate polyps. At least eight different genes have been identified in which mutations give rise to HNPCC. All these genes are involved in DNA mismatch repair. When both copies of the same mismatch repair gene are damaged, cells do not immediately proliferate to form polyps, as is seen in APC mutations, but are more prone to mutations that then lead to polyps. When this occurs, and polyps appear, the cells of these polyps have already acquired additional DNA damage and so are much more prone to further damage and hence to overt cancer. Thus, in this syndrome, there are few polyps, but a much higher proportion of them develop into malignant cancer. Sufferers from this syndrome have about a 75% chance of getting colon cancer.

Xeroderma pigmentosa

Xeroderma pigmentosa (XP) is very unusual because its pattern of inheritance is recessive (sufferers must inherit a defective copy of the gene from each parent). Since it is highly unlikely that two people, each carrying one defective copy of the same gene, would have a child together, XP is very rare.

Why should a mutation in one of the two copies of some genes (a dominant mutation) result in a high susceptibility to cancer, when in other cases both copies of the gene must be damaged (a recessive mutation)? The answer seems to lie in the mechanism by which the defect misdirects cell behaviour. In familial adenomatous polyposis or Li-Fraumeni syndrome, all the body's cells have one defective copy of a key gene; the loss of the remaining 'good' copy is enough to make that cell initiate a tumour. Therefore, inheriting one defective copy of such a gene will be enough to make that person prone to develop cancer. However, in XP, loss of both copies of a gene is not sufficient to initiate cancer; subsequent damage by a carcinogen is needed to initiate the cancer's development. In such a case, the chances of a person who has inherited just one defective copy of the gene developing cancer is not distinguishable from the risk for the general population.

Ataxia telangiectasia

Ataxia telangiectasia (AT) is also a recessive syndrome. Like XP, it is exceptionally rare, seen in less than 1 person in 100,000. In

AT, the mutated gene is involved in DNA repair. The protein encoded by the AT gene is believed to sense double-stranded breaks in DNA and activate the P53 pathway. AT patents are notably sensitive to the effects of ionising radiation, since this particularly causes double-strand breaks. An observation that led to the understanding of the mechanism of AT was that patients were hypersensitive to the X-rays used in treating their cancers.

The resulting genome instability makes AT carriers very prone to develop cancer of the blood and breast. About 40% of patients will develop cancer; many will develop more than one. It is not altogether surprising that blood cells are particularly susceptible, as double-strand breaks and incorrect re-joining of the broken ends is a particular feature of leukaemias. In AT-affected people, there is also a gradual loss of functional neurons in the cerebellum, causing rapid decline in co-ordination of movement and balance during childhood. This and a range of other defects mark the definitive features of this disease.

Glossary

Angiogenesis The growth of new blood vessels. In cancer, it is necessary for such vessels to penetrate the tumour to provide oxygen and nutrients.

Apoptosis The process by which cells kill themselves using energy and specialized cellular machinery. This allows cells to die without causing inflammation. See also *necrosis*.

Basal cell carcinomas A type of skin cancer that does not involve the pigment cells; common, but highly curable.

Bases See *DNA bases*.

Benign A tumour that does not have the ability to spread. Often reaches only a few millimetres in size, but some grow much larger.

Biopsy Analysis of a small piece of tissue taken from the living body to determine the presence, extent or stage of disease.

Bowel The long tubular region of the gut that runs from the stomach to the rectum, made up of the long (about 20 feet), narrow small intestine (small bowel) and the shorter (about 5 feet) and much broader large intestine (large bowel), which ends at the rectum. About 97% of colorectal cancers are in the large bowel or rectum with about 50% in the rectum or sigmoid colon (the last part before the rectum).

Brachytherapy Type of radiotherapy in which a solid source of radiation, that can only penetrate a short distance through tissues, is placed in the region of the tumour such that the tumour receives a continuous dose of radiation whilst most of the tissue is unaffected.

BRCA Tumour suppressor gene, derived from BReast CAncer. When mutated forms of either the BRCA1 or BRCA2 genes are inherited, women have a very high risk of developing breast or ovarian cancer.

Cancer Malignant proliferating cell population, means that the tumour can spread.

Cancer stem cell See *stem cell*.

Carcinogen Agent capable of causing cancer.

Carcinogenesis The process of cancer formation.

Caretaker A gene or its protein that plays a role in protecting DNA from damage, maintaining genomic integrity.

Caspases A family of enzymes that are able to digest other proteins into several pieces to help cells undergo the process of programmed cell death (apoptosis).

Catechins A family of chemicals making up part of the flavinol group of antioxidants. Found in green tea, but also in cocoa beans and prune juice.

CDK (Cyclin Dependent Kinase) Enzyme that act in partnership with the cyclins to control the cell cycle. 'Kinase' indicates that they function by adding phosphate groups to target proteins.

Cell cycle The processes that occur between one cell division and the next. Made up of a series of phases during which all the components of the cell are duplicated in a carefully co-ordinated fashion.

Centrosome Complex structure that is formed as the chromosomes prepare to separate into the two new daughter cells during cell division. They act as anchor points for the spindle that attaches to each chromosome and play a role in separating the chromosomes to either end of the mother cell before it divides in two.

Checkpoints Points in the cell cycle when the cycle can be halted in response to stress or DNA damage.

Chromosomes The large structures made up of DNA, packaged within various proteins to allow the huge length of DNA to fit into the nucleus of each cell. The human genome is shared between 23 pairs of these chromosomes, each pair carrying a different subset of genes.

Colonoscopy A medical procedure in which a thin, flexible tube carrying a video camera (a colonoscope) is inserted into the anus and passed up through the lower part of the bowel. The bowel is normally emptied for 1–2 days before the procedure using some form of laxative and patients often also receive a mild sedative to help them relax. The colonoscope can also be equipped to collect samples or remove polyps from the lining of the bowel.

Cyclin   Protein that is synthesized and degraded in a fluctuating manner coincident with the phases of the cell cycle. This cyclic rise and fall helps regulate the timing of the cell cycle.

Cytokinesis   The part of the cell cycle in which the mother cell physically divides into two new daughter cells.

Dendritic cell   Type of cell in the immune system that processes and presents alien proteins to the rest of the immune system to stimulate a response. Currently developed as a means to generate an immune response to tumours by immunization.

Differentiation   The process by which cells go from immature cells of an embryo or stem cells in adult tissues to mature specialized cell types, such as skin cells or neurons. This process also takes place in many tumours, such that the tumours contain both dividing immature cells and many non-dividing differentiated cells.

Differentiated   Description of a cell that has progressed to become a specialized, non-dividing cell, such as skin cells or neurons.

DNA   Deoxyribonucleic acid. The chemical material from which the genome (organized into chromosomes) is made.

DNA bases   Adenine (A), guanine (G), cytosine (C) and thymine (T), the parts of the DNA that vary along its length. The precise order of these bases represents the genetic code and not only allows different proteins to be made from different genes but also DNA to be replicated, producing new identical copies at each cell division.

DNA polymerase   The enzyme that synthesizes DNA.

Endothelium   Sub-type of epithelium (tightly associated layer of cells) that lines the internal surfaces of the heart, blood vessels and lymphatic system.

Epithelium   Tightly associated layer of cells that lines the internal and external surfaces of the body's organs, including skin, gut lining and endothelium of blood vessels.

Expression (gene)   When a gene is 'switched on', meaning that it is copied into RNA, where it is then usually translated into a protein.

Extracellular matrix   The complex mixture of large protein and sugar-based molecules that surrounds the cells in solid tissues.

Free radical   A very reactive molecule with an unpaired electron. Can be generated by carcinogens such as radiation; able to cause mutations by reacting with DNA.

Gatekeeper   A gene or its protein that plays a role in regulating the cell cycle in response to events that might cause cancer (include P53, Rb and APC).

Gene   Region within the DNA of a genome that codes for a protein.

Genome   The total DNA complement of a cell nucleus that makes up the entire chromosomal complement of a cell.

Growth factor   Protein that triggers a cascade of events leading to proliferation by binding to a receptor on the surface of a cell.

Hayflick limit   The number of cell divisions a particular cell can undergo before it becomes senescent, typically about 50.

Immune checkpoints   A series of signalling pathways in the cells of the immune system, that generally function to limit their activity and so avoid excess immune responses that might be damaging to the body. Cancer cells act via these pathways to avoid the attentions of the immune system and these have therefore become a target for drugs to activate the immune system to attack cancer cells.

Immunoediting   The process by which variant cancer cells arise within a tumour as a result of the immune system killing non-resistant cells. Very like Darwinian evolution, the selective pressure of the immune system selects for cells that are recognized less well by the immune system. The production of these less immunogenic variants is driven by the genetic variation between tumour cells due to the high levels of mutation seen within tumour cells.

Malignant   Describes a tumour able to spread locally or to other parts of the body; a tumour that has become cancerous because it can now metastasize.

Malignant melanoma   Aggressive form of skin cancer, composed of abnormal melanocytes.

Melanocytes   The pigmented cells of the skin.

Melanin   The pigment made by melanocytes that protects them from the damaging effects of ultraviolet radiation.

Mesothelioma   Cancer of the chest cavity, usually resulting from exposure to asbestos.

Metalloproteinases   Enzymes that can digest the matrix of protein and sugar surrounding cells (the extracellular matrix) to facilitate cell movement. Produced, for example, by the cells of the blood vessels when they grow.

Metastasis   The process by which cancer cells move from the primary tumour to secondary sites in other parts of the body.

Metastatic   A tumour that can spread to other parts of the body.

Mutagen   An agent that can cause mutations.

Mutation   A change in the sequence of bases of the DNA, which may (or may not) cause a change in the structure or function of the cell.

Mutagenesis   The process of generating mutations.

MYC   The gene that codes for the protein MYC, which acts as a transcription factor and is a powerful and frequently activated oncogene.

Necrosis   Cell death resulting from external damage or lack of oxygen. Unlike apoptosis, tends to result in local tissue inflammation.

Nucleotide   The sub-unit of DNA, made up of a five-carbon ribose sugar ring linked to both a base (A, G, C or T) and one or more phosphate groups.

Nucleus   The sub-cellular structure in which the DNA genome is stored and where the processes of DNA replication and transcription of the genes into RNA takes place.

Oncogene   A gene that encodes a protein that plays a part in initiating tumour formation when that gene is activated. This usually applies to a mutated or over-expressed version of that gene's normal counterpart. Although the normal gene is correctly called a 'proto-oncogene', the term oncogene is sometimes applied to both the normal and altered versions. Includes genes such as C–MYC and RAS.

P53   A tumour-suppressor gene that codes for a protein that can block the cell cycle and activate apoptosis.

Papilloma   A small benign tumour, such as a wart.

Pharmacogenomics   The science of linking the detailed sequence of a person's individual genome to their response to therapeutic drugs.

Polycyclic hydrocarbon   Type of carcinogen found in tobacco smoke and barbecued meat.

Polymerase   See *DNA polymerase*.

Polyp   Small outgrowth usually in gut; most are benign.

Polyposis   Disease state in which many polyps form.

Proliferation   The increase in numbers of cells through cell division.

Protein   Functional molecule produced from a gene. Includes enzymes, transcription factors, growth factors and many of the structural components of the cell.

Pyrimidine   General chemical term for the C and T bases that form part of the structure of DNA. G and C bases are called purines.

Pyrimidine dimers   Joining together of adjacent pyrimidine bases (C or T) in DNA caused by certain mutagens (especially ultraviolet radiation).

RAS   The gene or the protein it encodes; relays signals from cell surface receptors to other cellular components to tell the cells to divide. A powerful and frequently activated oncogene.

Rb   The gene and the tumour suppressor it encodes; can inhibit the cell cycle and trigger apoptosis, first discovered in the tumour of the eye, retinoblastoma.

Reactive oxygen species O_2^-, a form of oxygen that exists as a free radical and so is very reactive with other components of the cell. Generated by carcinogens such as radiation; able to cause mutations by reacting with DNA.

Recombination The process by which one region of a chromosome becomes joined to another to which it would not normally be attached, such as when a hybrid chromosome is produced linking part of one chromosome to part of another.

Retinoblastoma Tumour of the eye in which the tumour suppressor, Rb, was first discovered.

Ribosome The large multi-molecular complex that translates messenger RNA into proteins.

RNA Ribonucleic acid. The chemical (very similar to DNA in structure) that DNA is copied into, so that it can move out of the nucleus to be translated into protein.

Senescence The process of cellular ageing that limits the ability of normal cells to divide forever. Believed to be largely due to the gradual erosion of telomeres from the ends of the chromosomes.

Sigmoidoscopy A medical procedure very like a colonoscopy, but easier, and quicker. Like colonoscopy, a thin, flexible tube carrying a video camera (a colonoscope) is inserted into the anus and passed up through the lower part of the bowel. The bowel is normally emptied for 1–2 days before the procedure using some form of laxative. Unlike colonoscopy, no sedative is normally required, as the tube is only inserted a short way into the rectum and the very last part of the colon. As with the colonoscope, the tube can also be equipped to collect samples or remove polyps from the lining of the bowel.

Squamous cell carcinoma A type of skin cancer that does not involve the pigment cells; common, but highly curable.

Stem cell A cell that can undergo unlimited cell divisions and can typically give rise to several cell types. These include embryonic stem cells, only present in early embryos and capable of producing all cell types of the body. In adults, most tissues appear to harbour a small proportion of tissue-specific stem cells that can give rise to some or all of the cell types of that organ, such as blood or skin. The 'cancer stem cell', which is sometimes considered the same as the Tumour Initiating Cell or Tumour Propagating Cell, is a cell that can seed a new tumour, a feature that many cancer cells do not appear to possess. However, the abilities and precise definition of cancer stem cells is a much debated and hot topic of research.

Telomerase   Enzyme that can add telomeres to the ends of chromosomes, activated in many cancer cells.

Telomeres   Repeated structures at the ends of chromosomes that are gradually lost with each cell division. They are believed to provide protection from damage to more important DNA sequences and avoid the ends of the chromosomes being detected as broken DNA.

Template strand   One of the pair of strands of DNA that is copied to make a new matching strand during DNA replication. The template strand is the old strand that is used as a template for the new strand's synthesis.

Transcription   The process by which RNA is copied from DNA, as seen when a gene is expressed to produce its protein.

Transcription factor   A protein that controls whether a gene is expressed, thus determining if a protein is produced from that gene.

Translation   The process by which RNA is copied into protein.

Tumour   Abnormal growth of cells that can be either benign or malignant.

Tumour initiation   The process that starts tumour or cancer formation, often through mutation of an oncogene or a tumour suppressor. For cells to become fully developed cancers, they usually still need to undergo several more mutational events.

Tumour progression   The processes that cells go through as they develop from the initial start of tumour formation through to metastasis.

Tumour suppressor   A gene that plays a part in initiating tumour formation when it is *in*activated. Most tumour suppressors normally help to prevent cell division or promote apoptosis, so their mutation results in deregulation of these processes. Includes genes such as P53 and Rb.

Tyrosine kinase   An enzyme that can add a phosphate molecule to proteins at the amino acid, tyrosine. Many receptors at the cell surface have this enzymatic activity when they bind their specific signal molecule as it reaches the outside of the cell.

Further reading

Websites

For most readers, an up-to-date and accessible source of much information can be obtained from a wide range of websites. I have found none to match the site of the charity Cancer Research UK (www.cancerresearchuk.org). I am very grateful to those who created and maintain this site and provide an exceptionally valuable resource of information.

Related books

One in Three: A Son's Journey into the History and Science of Cancer by Adam Wishart (first edition published by Profile, 2006). Mixes passages on his experience of his father's battle with cancer with descriptions of the recent history of cancer research and some basic biology. A good read, providing valuable insight into the experience of having a relative with cancer and the history of cancer research, with some limited description of the biology of cancer.

Textbooks

Bruce Alberts et al., *Essential Cell Biology: An Introduction to the Molecular Biology of the Cell* (Garland Science). A simpler introductory text for newcomers to the field; written to provide a 'straightforward explanation of the workings of a living cell'.

Bruce Alberts et al., *Molecular Biology of the Cell* (Garland Science). The bible of cell biology for undergraduates and postgraduates.

Lewis J. Kleinsmith, *Principles of Cancer Biology* (Pearson Benjamin Cummings). Covers similar ground to Weinberg but is a shorter, lighter text.

F. Tannock, Richard P. Hill, Robert G. Bristow and Lea Harrington, *The Basic Science of Oncology* (McGraw Hill). Covers the same ground as Weinberg but in less detail. In addition, includes very detailed coverage of more clinically relevant issues, such as the mechanisms of therapy and epidemiology.

Robert A. Weinberg, *The Biology of Cancer* (Garland Science). Ideal text for science undergraduates or postgraduates studying cancer.

Jacob Wolff, *The Science of Cancerous Disease from Earliest Times to the Present* (Science History). First published in 1907. A very detailed and comprehensive description of published work relating to cancer, from Egyptian papyruses to the end of the nineteenth century.

Journal papers

Scientific American 18 (3) has a range of articles on cutting-edge aspects of cancer study.

1. A brief history of cancer

Rosalie David and Michael Zimmerman, Cancer: an old disease, a new disease or something in between. *Nature Reviews Cancer* 10, 2010, 728–733

2. The circle of life

R. Shackelford et al., Cell cycle control, checkpoint mechanisms and genotoxic stress. *Environmental Health Perspectives* 107, Supplement 1, 1999, 5–24

3. The immortal cell

R. Funayama and F. Ishikawa, Cellular senescence and chromatin structure. *Chromosoma* 116, 2007, 431–440

F.H. Igney and P.H. Krammer, Death and anti-death: tumour resistance to apoptosis. *Nature Reviews Cancer* 2, 2002, 277–288

S.A. Stewart and R.A. Weinberg (2006), Telomeres: cancer to human aging. *Annual Reviews in Cell and Developmental Biology* 22, 2006, 531–557

4. Surviving and spreading

A.F. Chambers et al., Dissemination and growth of cancer cells in metastatic sites. *Nature Reviews Cancer* 2, 2002, 563–572

A. Corthay, Does the immune system naturally protect against cancer? *Frontiers in Immunology*, 5, 2014, 197

L.M. Ellis and D.J. Hicklin, VEGF-targeted therapy: mechanisms of anti-tumour activity. *Nature Reviews Cancer* 8, 2008, 579–591

I.J. Fidler, The pathogenesis of cancer metastasis: the 'seed and soil' hypothesis revisited. *Nature Reviews Cancer* 3, 2002, 1–6

D.X. Nguyen et al., Metastasis: from dissemination to organ-specific colonisation. *Nature Reviews Cancer* 9, 2009, 274–284

Stephen Paget, The distribution of secondary growths in cancer of the breast. *The Lancet* 133, 1889, 571–573

5. *Mutation, mutation, mutation*

R. Shackelford et al., Cell cycle control, checkpoint mechanisms and genotoxic stress. *Environmental Health Perspectives* 107, Supplement 1, 1999, 5–24

6. *Chemical carcinogens*

P.J. Brooks et al., The alcohol flushing response: an unrecognized risk factor for esophageal cancer from alcohol consumption. *PLoS Medicine* 6, 2009, e1000050

Roger Collier, Health advocates assail Canada's asbestos stance. *Canadian Medical Association Journal* 179, 2008, 1257

P. Jha, Avoidable global cancer deaths and total deaths from smoking. *Nature Reviews Cancer* 9, 2009, 655–664

Laurie Kazan-Allen, Asbestos and mesothelioma: worldwide trends. *Lung Cancer* 49S1, 2005, S3–S8

M. López-Lµzaro, Anticancer and carcinogenic properties of curcumin: considerations for its clinical development as a cancer chemopreventative and chemotherapeutic agent. *Molecular Nutrition and Food Research* 52, 2008, S103–S127

Nature Outlook 513, Supplement S1-S48 Lung Cancer, 2014

R.N. Proctor, Tobacco and the global lung cancer epidemic. *Nature Reviews Cancer* 1, 2001, 82–86

G. Tweedale, Asbestos and its lethal legacy. *Nature Reviews Cancer* 2, 2002, 1–5

C.S. Yang et al. Cancer prevention by tea: animal studies, molecular mechanisms and human relevance. *Nature Reviews Cancer* 9, 2009, 429–439

7. Radiation

A.J. Miller and M.C. Mihm, Mechanisms of disease: melanoma. *New England Journal of Medicine* 355, 2006, 51–65

8. Catching cancer

M. Asaka, *Helicobacter pylori* infection and gastric cancer. *Internal Medicine* 41, 2002, 1–6

F.X. Bosch et al., Primary liver cancer: worldwide incidence and trends. *Gastroenterology* 127, 2004, S5–S16.

9. We are all different

V. Beral, Breast cancer and hormone-replacement therapy in the Million Women Study. *The Lancet* 362, 2003, 419–427

C. Turnbull and N. Rahman, Genetic predisposition to breast cancer: past, present and future. *Annual Review of Genomics and Human Genetics* 9, 2008, 321–345

10. Inheriting cancer

K. Hemminki et al. Genetic epidemiology of cancer: from families to heritable genes. *International Journal of Cancer* 111, 2004, 944–950

R. Shackelford et al., Cell cycle control, checkpoint mechanisms and genotoxic stress. *Environmental Health Perspectives* 107, Supplement 1, 1999, 5–24

C. Turnbull and N. Rahman, Genetic predisposition to breast cancer: past, present and future. *Annual Reviews in Genomics and Human Genetics* 9, 2008, 321–345.

11. It shouldn't happen to children

Paul J. Scotting et al. Children's solid tumours: a developmental disorder. *Nature Reviews Cancer* 5, 2005, 481–488

12. Attacking cancer

A. Anttila et al. Cervical cancer screening programmes and policies in 18 European countries. *British Journal of Cancer* 91, 2004, 935–941

NHS Choices, Breast cancer screening. Online at http://www.nhs.uk/Conditions/breast-cancer-screening/Pages/why-its-offered.aspx

N.J. West et al. Colorectal cancer screening in Europe: differences in approach; similar barriers to overcome. *International Journal of Colorectal Disease* 24, 2009, 731–740

13. Prevention and cure

M.H. Chang et al. Universal hepatitis B vaccination in Taiwan and the incidence of hepatocellular carcinoma in children. *New England Journal of Medicine* 336, 1997, 1855–1859

Andy Coghlan, Cancer's penicillin moment: drugs that unleash the immune system. *New Scientist* 3063, 5 March 2016

Francis S Collins and Anna D Barker, Mapping the cancer genome. *Scientific American* 18, 2008, 22–29

C. Coyle, F.H. Cafferty and R.E. Langley, Aspirin and colorectal cancer prevention and treatment: is it for everyone? *Current Colorectal Cancer Reports* 12, 2016, 27–34

L.M. Ellis and D.J. Hickling, VEGF-targeted therapy: mechanisms of anti-tumour activity. *Nature Reviews Cancer* 8, 2008, 579–591

F.J. Esteva and G.N. Hortobagyi, Gaining ground on breast cancer. *Scientific American* 18, 2008, 88–96

K. Imai and A. Takaoka, Comparing antibody to small-molecule therapies for cancer. *Nature Reviews Cancer* 6, 2006, 714–727

C.J. Melief, Cancer immunotherapy by dendritic cells. *Immunity* 29, 2008, 372–383

L.J. Old, Cancer vaccines: an overview. *Cancer Immunity*, Supplement 1, 2008, 1–4

D.M. Parkin, L. Boyd and L.C. Walker, The fraction of cancer attributable to lifestyle and environmental factors in the UK in 2010: Summary and conclusions. *British Journal of Cancer* 105, 2011, S77-S81

R. Roden and T.C. Wu, How will HPV vaccines affect cervical cancer? *Nature Reviews Cancer* 6, 2006, 753–763

E. Szabo, Selecting targets for cancer prevention: where do we go from here? *Nature Reviews Cancer* 6, 2006, 867–874

US Preventative Services Task Force: *Aspirin Use to Prevent Cardiovascular Disease and Colorectal Cancer: Preventive Medication. Online at http://www. uspreventiveservicestaskforce.org/Page/Document/RecommendationStatement-Final/aspirin-to-prevent-cardiovascular-disease-and-cancer*

Index

acute lymphoblastic leukaemia
(ALL) *118*
adenoma 119
Africa
AIDS *90*
Epstein-Barr virus
infection 91–2
hepatitis infection 92
age
and cervical cancer 93–4, 162
distribution of cancers *124*
and life expectancy 11
and lung cancer 67–8
and prostate cancer 110, 139
and UK screening for breast,
cervical and bowel/
colorectal cancer 136–42
and women developing breast
cancer 104, 121
see also children; young people
age-related macular
degeneration 159
AIDS (acquired immune deficiency
syndrome) *90*, 193
alcohol
defective gene for breakdown
of 73
and increased risk of breast
cancer 109
role in cancer risk 168–9, 171,
176
types of cancer caused by *60*
alkylating agents 66

amino acids 20
anaemia 148
Ancient Egypt, earliest recorded
description of cancer 6–7
androgen ablation 157
angiogenesis 40–1, 199
anti-angiogenetic therapies 159
antibiotics 95
antibodies
immune system 49–50
in new biological
therapies 156, 159–60
see also herceptin; monoclonal
antibodies; immunoediting
apoptosis (process of cell death) 31,
34–8, 48, 144–5, 199
cancer cells' evasion of 37–8
archaeology, evidence of cancer
sufferers 7–8
aromatase inhibitors 156–7
asbestos
as cause of mesothelioma *60*,
65, 69–70
exposure to 69
production and trade 70–1
asbestosis 69
Asia *see* Southeast Asia
aspirin 169–71
ataxia telangiectasia (AT) *118*,
197–8
atomic bombs 84–5
atoms 77, 83
Aulus Cornelius Celsus 8

Australia
  banning of asbestos 68
  high rates of skin cancer 81
  autopsy, and developments in
    understanding of cancer 8–9

babies
  pre-leukaemic cells 126
  cancer free, PGD 177–8
  see also embryos
bacteria
  and antibiotics used in cancer
    drugs 147
  H. pylori and association with
    cancer 90, 95–6
Barr, Yvonne 91
basal cell carcinomas 78, 199
benign tumours 3, 27, 33, 55–8,
    79, 93, 195, 199
  see also adenoma; moles; polyps
biological therapies
  activating the immune
    system 159–63
  impact of human genome
    analysis 151, 164, *164–5*
  successful developments 109,
    155–8
  targets for new
    treatments 158–9
biopsy 139, 199
black populations, low incidence
    of skin cancer 80
bladder cancer 60, 66, *105*, 167
bleomycin 147
blood cancers
  predisposition syndrome *118*,
    198
  see also leukaemias

blood cells
  replenished by stem cells 149
  see also anaemia; dendritic
    cells; immune system;
    lymphocytes
blood tests, screening for
    cancer 166–7
blood vessels
  in age-related macular
    degeneration 159
  cancer's need for nourishment
    from 39–41, 159
  cells' penetration into 45–6
bone cancer 7, *118*, 129, 166, 195
bone marrow
  severe side effects in 148–9
  transplantation 149
bowel cancer 72–3, 75, *105*, *118*
  screening for 140–2, 205
  see also colorectal cancer
brachytherapy 145–6, 199
brain tumours *105*, 174, 194,
    196
  predisposition syndromes *118*,
    177, 194–8
  problematic nature of
    surgery 143
  treatment of children 129, 131
BRCA genes *118*, 120–1, 177,
    199
breast cancer *105*
  benefits from new biological
    therapies 155–8
  as biggest cause of women's
    cancer deaths 67
  carcinogens causing *60*
  and defective genes 120–1
  dietary factors reducing
    risk 73, 75

breast cancer (*cont.*):
  early diagnosis and unnecessary
    surgery *137–8*
  and family inheritance of
    genes 120–1
  in historical descriptions of
    cancer 7–9, 13
  hormones and women's risk
    of 104–7
  and HRT risk 107–9
  inheriting cancer
    predisposition syndromes *118*,
    120–1, 177
  in men 110
  as most common cancer in
    UK *105*
  pharmacogenomics
    approaches 163–4
  potential of drugs for
    preventive treatment 168–9
  role of alcohol in causing 73
  secondary tumours from 46
  use of antibodies in new
    targeting therapy 158–9
  X-ray mammography
    screening for 136–8
Breasted, James Henry 7
breastfeeding 13, 106–7
Britain *see* United Kingdom (UK)
Burkitt's lymphoma 91, 192

Canada 70–1
cancer predisposition
  syndromes 113–23, 194–8
Cancer Research UK *80*, 82,
  105, *111*, 175, 207
cancer stem cells *see* stem cells
capillaries and formation of
  secondary tumours 46, 48

carcinogens 6, 9–12, *60*, 65–89
  causing damage to DNA 62,
    166
  and children's cancers 121
  different responses to 101–3
  genes and susceptibility
    to 102–3
  variations in different parts of
    the world. 63–4
  see also chemical carcinogens;
    radiation; smoking;
    ultraviolet light
carcinomas 42, 199
caspases 36–7, 200
CAT scan 142
cats, feline leukaemia virus 95
CDK (cyclin dependent
  kinases) *184*, 185–7
cell cycle 23–5, *24*, *26*, 101,
  103, 181–6, *184*, 200
controls and checkpoints 23–6,
  28–9, 36, 186–8, *184*, 200
cell death
  in chemotherapy and
    radiotherapy 144–5
  see also apoptosis
cell division 17–18, *19*
  damage and mutations 27–9,
    55–6, 130
  and decay of
    chromosomes 31–3
  DNA replication 22–3, *22*,
    18, 55, 181–3, *182*
  impact of chemotherapy and
    radiotherapy 147–51
  importance of MYC protein
    for 188–9
  key role of APC gene 195
  and stem cells 158–9
  see also proliferation of cells

centrosomes 183–4
cerebellum
   brain tumours in children 129
   loss of neurons caused by AT
      syndrome 198
cervical cancer *105*
   association with age 93–4
   carcinogens causing *60*
   and contraceptive pill 107
   HPV virus causing *90*, 93,
      162, 193
   screening for 138–9
   and sexual activity 93–4
   vaccination programmes 139,
      162
chemical carcinogens 64, 65
   asbestos *60*, 69–71, 203
   in diet *60*, 71–75
   tobacco smoke *60*, 66–9
chemical castration 156
chemotherapy 137, 146–7
   accompanying surgery 143
   compared with
      radiotherapy 150
   induction of apopotosis 37
   new biological therapies
      combined with 157
   principle behind 143
   side-effects 147–51
   testicular cancer 110
   see also combination
      chemotherapy
Chernobyl disaster (1986) 86,
   144
children
   leukaemias 127
   occurrence of cancer in 124–5,
      124
   solid tumours in 127–30
   treating cancer in 130–2

China
   hepatitis infection 92
   increase in smokers 68
chromosomes 29, *57*, 200
   behaviour in leukaemias 126–9
   in cell cycle 23–4, 183–4,
      187, 200
   effects of damaged DNA 56–7,
      57, 129
   effects of vincristine on 147
   gradual shortening and
      decay of 31–3, 205–6
   inheritance of *19*, 22–23, *22*
   recombination 33–4
   see also DNA
      (deoxyribonucleic acid)
circulatory system, role in spread
      of tumour 39–42, 45–6
clinical trials 74, 153, 155,
   157–8, 160–3, 165
colon cancer
   and the contraceptive pill 107
   carcinogens causing *60*
   dietary factors *60*, 72–4
   geographical distribution 64
   and HRT 108
   in identical twins 102
   inheriting predisposition
      syndromes *118*, 119–20,
      171–2, 195–7
   polyps progressing to 56, 58,
      119, 195, 196–7
   screening 140–2, 166–7
   secondary tumours arising
      from 46
colonoscopy 140–2, 166, 200,
   205
combination chemotherapy 148
computerised tomography *see*
      CAT scan

contraceptive pill 107, 109
CT colonography 142
curcumin 73–74
Curie, Irène 86
Curie, Marie 86
cyclins 185–6, 200
CYPs 72, 106
Cytochrome P450 72
cytokinesis 183–4, 186, 201
cytology test 139

Dally, Clarence 86
Darwin, Charles 56
Deaths 42, 153
    and aspirin protective
        effects 170–1
    from breast cancer 104, 121
    from cancer caused by
        asbestos 70
    from lung cancer 59, 66–8, 88
    from cancer caused by diet 72
    cancer caused by different
        infectious agents 90
    cervical cancer cases 93
    cervical cancer vaccination and
        prevention of 162
    cervical screening and
        reduction of 138–9
    from children's cancer 125
    from colon cancer 142
    from different classes of disease
        154
    estimates of annual number
        caused by cancer 60
    due to inherited
        predispositions 117
    from liver cancer 92
    recent fall in deaths from
        cancer 153

    from skin cancers caused by
        sunlight 79, 81
    from stomach cancer 96
deep-vein thrombosis 158
dendritic cells 162, 201
designer babies 177
developed countries
    HPV virus and association
        with cancer 93
    testicular cancer 110
    trends increasing risk of breast
        cancer 107
developing countries
    increase in smokers 68
    and potentially avoidable
        cancers 96
    risk of developing liver
        cancer 92
    use of asbestos 70
    viruses associated with
        cancer 92
diet
    factors causing cancers 60,
        71–5
    factors reducing risk of
        cancers 96, 168, 172–3,
        175, 176
    and increased risk of breast
        cancer 109, 138
    of monks of Mount Athos
        monasteries 71, 91
differentiated cells 17, 201
DNA (deoxyribonucleic
    acid) 21, 201
    adducts advances in analysis
        of 164
    bases 19, 20–1, 21, 65–6, 164,
        181, 190, 199, 201, 203–4
    changes caused by chemical
        carcinogens 65

damage by chemotherapy 150
damage and mutations
  affecting machinery of 13,
  18, 27–9, 31–4, 36–7, 55–7,
  59, 66, 121–3, 128–30,
  185–8, 190, 194, 197, 200
damage by radiation/
  radiotherapy and
  chemotherapy 78, 79–80,
  144–5, 150,174
and detection using blood and
  urine tests 167
errors occurring during repair
  process 62–3, 84
impact of chemotherapy agents
  on 144–5, 150
inheritance of mistakes and
  mutations 61, 114–6, 117,
  127
nucleotide 19, 190, 203
polymerase 181, 190–1, 201
repair of 24–5, 121-2, 187,
  190-1, 196-8
replication process and
  children's cancer 128–9
structure 19, 20
synthesis 19, 20, 23–4, 27–8,
  128–31, 181–3, 182, 186,
  206
template strand 190, 206
transcription of 20, 21, 203,
  206
see also cell division;
  chromosomes; genes;
  genome; recombinant DNA
  technology
Drosophila melanogaster (fruit
  fly) 44
drugs 146–7
  current clinical trials in US 153

and pharmacogenomics 163–5,
  204
and problems in development
  for children's cancers 132
used in biological
  therapies 155–63

Eastern Europe 95
E-cadherin 42–3
e-cigarettes 68
Edison, Thomas 86
Edwin Smith Papyrus see Smith,
  Edwin
egg cells, genes 116
embryos
  losses due to genetic
    abnormalities 128
  screening of 177
emphysema 66
endometrial cancer 108, 118,
  158
endothelial cells 40–1, 47
environmental carcinogens 109,
  113, 128
environmental risk factors, breast
  cancer 106, 109
EPIC (European Prospective
  Investigation into
  Cancer) 72–3
epithelial tissues, carcinomas
  derived from 42, 43
Epstein, Anthony 91
Epstein-Barr virus (EBV) 90,
  91–2, 95, 192
etoposide (chemotherapeutic) 17
Europe 72
  and Chernobyl disaster 86
  risk of developing lung
    cancer 88

Europe (*cont.*):
  and skin cancer 81–2
  study of prostate screening 140
  see also Eastern Europe
evolution process 51, 56, 202
Ewing, James 46, 48
Exercise *138*, *169*, 173, *176*
extracellular matrix 41, 45, 202, 203
eyes *see* age-related macular degeneration; retinoblastoma

faecal occult blood test (FOBT) 140–1
familial adenomatous polyposis *118*, 119, 195–6
Far East 64, 68, 95
  see also China; Japan; Korea
feline leukaemia virus 95
foetuses 128, 177
Folkman, Judah 40
food
  red meat 71–2, 75, 96, 171, *176*
  toxins as carcinogens 65, 69, 71–2
  types of cancer caused by *60*
  see also diet
Fraumeni, Joseph *see* Li-Fraumeni syndrome
free radicals 74–5, 83, 202, 205
  generated by radiotherapy 145
  and radiation-induced DNA damage *78*, 83, 145
Fuchs, Ernst 47

Galen (Claudius Galenus) 8
Gardner, Eldon J. 119, 195

gastritis 95
gatekeeper genes/proteins 24, 27, 187, 202
genes 2, 6, 178, 202
  affected by familial cancer syndromes *118*
  cells' inheritance of 22–3, *22*, 61, 119, 197
  evolution and variation in sequences 101–2
  expression 20, *21*, 202
  inheritance and predisposition to cancer 113–123
  names *44*
  protective against cancer 101–3
  viral 192
  see also human genome; mutations; oncogenes; tumour suppressor genes
genetic make-up
  and cancer predisposition 113
  and different responses to carcinogens 102–3
  and tailoring of individual therapies 163, 178
genetic screening 177
genitalia, and cancer *à deux* 10–11
genome 18, *19*,103, 200, 201, 202
  abnormality due to damaging mutations 56, *57*, 59, 61–3, 65, 68–9, 83, 129–30
  of cancer cells damaged by therapies 144, 146–7, 150
  replication in cell division 18, 23, 61, 147, 181–3, *182*, 187
  sequencing of 151, *164–5*, 178
  see also DNA (deoxyribonucleic acid); genes

geological features, release of radon gas 87

glandular fever *see* mono (infectious mononucleosis)

glioblastoma (brain tumour) 194

global warming 82

glutathione S-transferase 75

Greece *see* Mount Athos

green tea 73–4, 172–3, 200

growth factors 24, 149, 188, 204

GSTs *see* glutathione S-transferase

Gut 199
  and C-MYC gene 188
  and severity of side-effects from therapies 148, 150

hair loss 148

Hayflick limit 30, *32*, 202

health education/schemes *see* public health education/ schemes

hedgehog gene *44*

Helicobacter pylori (H. pylori) bacterium *90*, 95–6

hepatitis viruses *90*, 96, 161, 192–3
  vaccination against 92

HER2 156

herbicides 173

herceptin 156

hereditary cancer *see* cancer predisposition syndromes; family; genetic make-up

hereditary non-polyposis colon cancer (HNPCC) *118*, 119–20, 196–7

herpes virus 195

heterocyclic amines 72

Hieronymus Fabricius 8

Hiroshima 144
  survivors of atomic bomb 84–6

HIV (human immunodeficiency virus) 84–6

hormonal deprivation therapy *see* androgen ablation

hormones
  and breast cancer 103–9
  men and development of cancer 110–12
  and new biological therapies 155–6
  oestrogen 106–9
  progesterone 106–9
  prolactin 106
  testosterone and prostate cancer 110–12
  women and development of cancer 103

HRT (hormone replacement therapies)influence on cancer risk 107–9, *169*

human genome *see* genome

Human Papilloma Virus (HPV) *90*, 93–4, 107, *169*, 193
  vaccination against 96, 162

IAPs (inhibitors of apoptosis) 36–7

imaging techniques 135, 142, 166

immune surveillance 50

immune system antibodies 125–6, 154
  antibodies as therapeutic agents 154, 156–7, 159–60

immune system antibodies (*cont.*):
   association with cancers caused
      by Epstein–Barr virus 91–2
   effect of chemotherapy on 149
   effects of HIV on 94–5, 193
   failure to deal with cancer 49
   and leukaemias 126
   immunisation,
      successful vaccination
         programmes 161–3
immunoediting 51, 160, 202
in vitro fertilisation 177
infants *see* babies; children
infectious diseases
   and 'catching' cancer 10–11,
      64, 90–7, *90*, 162 *see also*
      viruses
inflammation 37, 199, 203
   and aspirin
   caused by asbestos 69
   caused by viruses 92, 192–3
   by *H. pylori* bacterium 95
inheritance
   of dominant and recessive
      mutations *114–16*, 117
   of genes 22–3, *22*
   risk of breast cancer 120–1
inherited predispositions
      to cancer *see* cancer
      predisposition syndromes
ipilimumab 160–1
Italy 8, 162

Japan 64, 70, 73, 89

Kaposi's sarcoma *90*, 193
kidney, cancer of *60*, 66, 75,
   105, 129

kidney transplants 50
Korea 73, 92
Kraske, Paul 4

lapatinib (biological therapy) 156
larynx, cancer of *60*, 168
leukaemias *105*
   and C-MYC gene 188
   carcinogens causing *60*, 66
   in children 125–6, 174–5
   predisposition syndromes *118*
   radiation's particular effect
      on 85–6
   risk for ataxia telangiectasia
      sufferers 198
   risk for Li-Fraumeni syndrome
      sufferers 194
   stem cell treatment and bone
      marrow replacement
      149–50
   use of imatanib in new
      treatment for 157
   see also blood cancers
Li-Fraumeni syndrome 117,
   118, 177, 194
life expectancy 11
lifestyle
   and avoidance of cancers 71,
      93, 96, 105, 153, 168,
      171–3, 175, *176*
   and women's risks of
      developing cancers 107–9,
      138
Litvinenko, Alexander 87
Liver 72, *105*
   secondary tumours in 46
   transplants 50
liver cancer
   in Asian people 64

carcinogens causing *60*, 66
in children 129
link with hepatitis virus *90*,
92, 162, 192
role of alcohol in causing 73
screening of blood and urine
for 167
side effects of therapy 161
surgery 142–3
use of antibodies in new
therapies for 159
LMP1 192
lung cancer *105*
carcinogens causing *60*
caused by asbestos 69
caused by radon gas 87–8
fall in smoking and decline
in 67
metastasis of breast cancer cells
and 166
mutations in genome 165
in predisposition
syndromes *118*, 194
rapid rise in 8–9, 68
as rare in children 127
rates compared with breast
cancer 104
secondary tumours in 46–7
smoking as main cause
of 66–8
use of new therapies for 157,
159, 161
lymph system, role in spread of
cancer 45–6
lymphocytes affected by
viruses 91, 192, 193
lymphocytic tumours 146
lymphomas *90*, 91,*105*,
192–3
see also Burkitt's lymphoma

macular degeneration *see* age-
related macular degeneration
Mad and Bub 187
malaria, co-infection with
Epstein-Barr virus 91
malignant melanoma *80*, 81, *105*,
203
caused by ultraviolet
radiation *60*, 78–9, *78*, 82,
165
geographical variation in
incidence of *80*
moles progressing to 33, 79, *79*
new therapies for 160–1, 163
malignant tumours 28, 41, 56
analysis showing distorted
chromosomes 57–8, *57*
mammography screening 136–8
Marshall, Barry 95
Massagué, J. 166
mechlorethamine 146
medulloblastoma (brain
tumour) 196
melanin 80–1, 103, 203
melanocytes 103, 203
men
hormones and cancer 102–4
lung cancer mortality rates 67
percentage developing
prostate cancer 57, 71, 110,
111
UK deaths from prostate
cancer *111*
menopause 109, 156
see also HRT (hormone
replacement therapies)
mesothelioma *60*, 69–70, 203
metalloproteinases 41, 45, 203
metastasis 42–51, *43*, 166, 203
see also secondary tumours

micro-organisms
  caused by bacteria *90*, 95–6,
    146
  types of cancer associated
    with *60*, *90*
  viruses 10, 50, 64, 90–5, *90*,
    139, 162, 192–3
microtubules 147
mitomycin 146
mitotic catastrophe 144–5
molecules *see* free radicals; small
    molecules
moles 31, 58
  progression towards malignant
    melanoma 79
mono (infectious
  mononucleosis) 85, 168
monoclonal antibodies 154
Morgagni, Giovanni Batista 8–9
Mount Athos, monks 71
mouth cancer *60*, 66, 73, 168
muscular dystrophies *114*
mutagenesis 128, *165*, 203
mutations 2, *44*, 55–64, 91
  in BRCA genes 120–1, 177
  cancer cells resistant to
    therapy 151
  in cancer progression 26–7
  caused by screening and
    therapy 144, 146, 150–1
  causes of 59, 62, 65–9, 77,
    85–6, 174
  causing immortality of cancer
    cells 31–3
  in cell cycle 56
  in children's solid
    cancers 127–30
  detected in new screening
    strategies 167
  and DNA repair 28, 56, 63, 190

disruption of DNA
    sequence 65–6, 203
dominant and recessive *114–6*,
    117
increased rate in cancers 28–9,
    57–9
inherited 113–23, *114–16*,
    118, 194–8
insights since sequencing of
    cancer genome 164, *164–5*
in leukaemias 125–6
and odds of getting cancer
    58–9
outside and within genes 62
P53, 28, 33–4, 37–8, 187, 194
and screening to avoid
    inheritance of 168, 177
tendency of infected cells to
    acquire 91, 193
MYC 188–9, 203, 204

Nagasaki 144
  survivors of atomic bomb
    84–5
  nasopharyngeal cancer *90*, 91,
    192
nausea 130, 148, 175
nervous system, cancers of *118*
neuroblastoma 131
neurofibromatosis *118*
neutropenia 149
nitrogen mustard 146
nivolumab 160–1
Nobel Prize 86, 95
North America 87, 92, 141
  see also Canada; United States
    of America (USA)
nuclear bombs 85–5
  see also atomic bombs

nuclear power plants *see*
    Chernobyl disaster (1986)
nuclear waste 77
nuns 93, 105

obesity
    and increase in risk of
        developing cancers 75, 109,
        173
    types of cancer caused by *60*
oesophagus, cancer of *60*, 66,
    73, 75, *105*, 168
oestrogen 100, 101
    in earlier treatment for prostate
        cancer 156
    and new biological therapies
        for breast cancer 155–6,
        158, 163
oncogenes 25–7, 30, 41, 126,
    203, 304
    carried by viruses 94, 193
    MYC protein 203
    1000 Genomes project *164*
Opvido™ 160
ovarian cancer *105*
    and HRT 108
    inheritance of 121, 199
ovarian suppression, used in
    therapies for breast cancer 156
ovulation 106

P53 (tumour suppressor gene/
    protein) 41, 204, 206
    and Ataxia telangiectasia 198
    and Human Papilloma
        Virus 94, 193
    and Li-Fraumeni
        syndrome 117, *118*, 194

mutations 28–9, 33, 37–8,
    145
    protective role in cell
        cycle 25, 32, 36, 144, *184*,
        185, 187–8, 202
Paget, Stephen 47–9
pancreas cancer *105*
    causes of *60*, 66, 75
    predisposition syndromes *118*,
        194
Pap smear 138–9
Paul of Aegina 8
pertuzumab (biological
    therapy) 156
pesticides 173–4
pharmaceutical companies 132
pharmacogenomics 163–4, 204
physiology 110, 112, 170
    and different responses to
        carcinogens 101
    and tailoring individual
        therapies 163
plant products used in
    chemotherapeutics 146–7
polonium 83
polycyclic hydrocarbons 66, 204
Polynesia 95
Polyphenols 74
polyposis 119, 204
    see also familial adenomatous
        polyposis
polyps 58, 204
    and colorectal cancer 119–20,
        140–1, 195–7, 201, 205
Pott, Percivall 10
pregnancy
    historical changes 13
    loss of embryos during 128
    and sex hormones, protective
        factor for breast cancer 106

prevention 168–73, *176*, 178
  aspects of diet 74
  development of therapeutic
    drugs for 153
  new screening strategies 166–7
  screening of embryos 177–8
  use of anti-cancer drugs 168–9
  use of aspirin 169–71
  vaccination programmes 161–3
progesterone 106–9
proliferation of cells 35, 56, 110,
    106–9, 204
  in children's cancers 129–30
  effect of inflammation
    on 69–70
  effect of viral genes on 91,
    192–3
  and formation of cancer 18,
    27, 33
  growth factors 149, 157, 188,
    202
  inhibitors 37, 146
  and polyps 195
  and women's hormonal
    surges 106, 155
prostate cancer 57, 71, *105*, *111*,
    178
  dietary factors reducing risk of
    73
  in identical twins 102
  predisposition syndrome
    associated with *118*
  provenge therapy 163
  screening for 136, 139–40
  targeting hormone-dependent
    cancer cells 156
  world-wide incidence 110,
    111
prostate specific antigen
    (PSA) 139–40, 167

proteins 20, 23, 55, 202, 204, 205
  effects of changes in DNA
    strands 28, 62
  encoded by genes 20, *21*, 25,
    114
  as markers for presence of
    cancers 167
  in replication of DNA 24, 61,
    185–7
  tumour associated antigens 50
  see also antibodies; cyclins;
    enzymes; transcription
    factors
proteomic analysis 167
proton beam therapy 145
provenge therapy 163
public health
  education/schemes to avoid
    infection by hepatitis B and
    C viruses 92
  and avoidance of cancers 96
  HPV vaccination 139, 161–2
  new screening strategies 166–7
pulmonary embolism 158
pyrimidine dimers 77, *78*, 204

radiation 64, 77–89, 169, 198
  from atomic bombs 84–5
  damage to DNA *78*, 83, 86
  day-to-day exposure and
    avoidance of 86–8
  ionising 77, 83
  used in radiotherapy 142,
    144–6
  see also ultraviolet light
radioisotopes 87, 144, 145–6
radiotherapy 135, 143
  brachytherapy 145–6, 199
  fractionation 145

improvements in 135, 150
principle behind 143
proton beam therapy 145
side-effects 131, 145, 147–8,
    150
in treatment of testicular
    cancer 110
radon 87–8
types of cancer caused by *60*
raloxifene 158, 168
RAS 188, 204
Rb
    gene/protein 25, *118*, 204,
        205, 206
    and Human Papilloma
        Virus 94, 193
    mutations 186, 188
    protective role in cell cycle 25,
        32, *184*, 185, 186, 188, 202
reactive oxygen species 83, 205
recombinant DNA
    technology 13
red blood cells *see* anaemia
red meat 71–2, 171
    avoidance of 75, 96, *176*
red-haired people 103
retina, cancer of, predisposition
    syndrome *118*
retinoblastoma 25, *118*, 204, 205
    see also Rb
    gene/protein ribonucleic acid
        see RNA
    RNA (ribonucleic acid) 20,
        21, 202, 205, 206
Ruskin, John 4
Russia, asbestos industry 70

Scandinavia 87
    see also Denmark

screening 135, 136–142
    and bowel cancer 140–2
    for BRCA1 and BRCA2
        mutations and breast
        cancer 121, 136–7, *137–8*
    for cervical cancer 139–40
    and exposure to radiation 88
    and liver cancer 92
    new, less invasive
        methods 166–7
scrotum, cancer of *see* 'soot-wart'
sebaceous cysts 195
secondary tumours 42, 45–8,
        143, 150, 203
    see also metastasis
senescence 31–4, 205
sex-specific cancers *105*
sexual behaviour/intercourse
    and avoidance of cancer 93
    and cervical cancer 93–4
side-effects 147
    chemotherapy 146, 148
    in children 130–2
    radiotherapy 145–6, 148–50
    in biological therapies 151,
        155, 158, 160–1, 169
sigmoidoscopy 141–2, 205
skin cancers avoidance of 80
    caused by exposure to
        sunlight 12, 77
    common occurrence of 78–9
    inheritance of 121–2
    non-melanoma forms 78
    predisposition syndrome *118*
    sensitivity of red-haired
        people 103
    see also malignant melanomas
skin tags 58
Sloan Kettering Cancer
        Centre 46

slug and snail genes/proteins 43, *44*
small molecules 154, 155, 161
  erlotinib 157
  imanatib (or glivec/gleevec) 157
  see also tamoxifen
smear test *see* Pap smear
Smith, Edwin, and Edwin Smith Papyrus 6, 7
smoking
  and added exposure to radon 88
  causing mutations in genome 165
  giving up and avoidance of cancer 96, 168, *176*
  and lung cancer rates 9
  as major cause of cancer 59, *60*, 66–8, *169*
snail gene/protein *see* slug and snail genes/proteins
'soot-wart' (cancer of the scrotum) 10
South America 95
Southeast Asia
  Epstein-Barr virus infection 91
  hepatitis infection 92
  see also Taiwan
  lung cancer in women 68–9
Soviet Union, Chernobyl disaster 86, 144
sperm cell divisions 116
squamous cell carcinomas 78, 205
stem cells 149–50, 158–9, 200, 205–6
stomach cancer *105*
  carcinogens causing *60*, 66
  diet as cause of 72
  high incidence in Japan 64

in identical twins 102
involving infection by *H. pylori* bacterium *90*, 95–6
predisposition syndrome *118*
secondary tumours arising from 46
stomach ulcers 95
stroke 158
sunbeds 82
sunlight *see* ultraviolet light; Xeroderma Pigmentosa (XP)
superoxide dismutase 75
surgery 42, 120, 142–3, 152
  and controversy over cancer screening 137, *137–8*, 140
  increased effectiveness of 135

Taiwan 73, 92, 161–2
tamoxifen 155, 157–8, 168
teas, inhibiting of tumour formation 73–4, 172–3, 200
telomerase *32*, 34, 206
telomeres *32*, 34, 206
teratocarcinoma 129
testicular cancer 110
  predisposition syndrome *118*
testosterone and prostate cancer 111, 156–7
therapies
  cancer cells resistant to 145, 149, 151, 155–6, 159, 166
  developments in treatment of children 132
  see also biological therapies; chemotherapy; drugs; pharmacogenomics; radiotherapy

thrombosis *see* deep-vein
   thrombosis
tobacco smoking *see* smoking
topoisomerase 147
toxins
   food 71–2, 74
   released by bacteria in *H.*
      pylori 95
   used in chemotherapy 148
transcription, in gene
      expression 20, *21*, *26*, 203,
      206
transcription factors 43, 188,
      203, 204, 206
translation, in gene
      expression *21*, *26*, 206
treatments *see* biological
      therapies; chemotherapy;
      drugs; radiotherapy;
      therapies
tumour suppressor genes 25,
      26–7, 30, 41, 94, 113, 206
   see also BRCA genes; P53, Rb,
      retinoblastoma
Turcots syndrome 196
twins, identical 102
tyrosine kinases 157

Ukraine *see* Chernobyl disaster
      (1986)
ultraviolet light
   exposure of humans to 12, 59,
      80–2, 88
   inducing mutations in
      genome 77, *165*, 204
   types of cancer caused by *60*,
      81
United Kingdom (UK)
   aspirin trial 170–1

avoidable cancers 168, *169*
bowel/colon cancer 64, 72,
      140–2
breast cancer statistics *104*,
      105, 107
cervical cancer 93–4, 162
common occurrence of skin
      cancers 12, 78–9, *80*, 81
deaths from skin cancers
      caused by sunlight 79
use of e-cigarettes 68
number of cancer deaths
      caused by smoking 66–7
obesity and cancer 75
proton beam therapy 145
radon exposure and lung
      cancer 88
screening embryos 177
screening for breast
      cancer 136
study to identify markers for
      breast cancer 167
United States of America
      (USA) 13, 46, 64, 175
age-related macular
      degeneration 159
breast cancer 109, 120
current clinical trials for
      treatments 153
deaths due to asbestos 70
deaths from skin cancers
      caused by sunlight 79
high occurrence of colon
      cancer 64
inherited colon cancers 119
number of people smoking 67
number of cancer deaths
      caused by smoking 59, 69
prostate cancer 140, 163
proton beam therapy 145

United States of America (*cont.*):
  screening for Li–Fraumeni
    syndrome 177
  sunbeds 82
  see also North America
urine tests 166–7
uterus, cancer of 8, 75, 107–8,
  105
  predisposition syndrome *118*
  see also endometrial cancer

vaccination 96, 161, 162
  against cervical cancer 92, 162
  against hepatitis B and C
    viruses 92, 162
  against HPV infections 94,
    139, 162
VEGF 41, 51, 159
vincristine 147
viruses
  and immunisation as weapon
    against cancers 96, 162, *176*
  playing role in causing
    cancer 55, 64, 90–6, *90*,
    139, 192–3
vitamins 74, 172

white blood cells depletion due
  to chemotherapy 149
  see also dendritic cells;
    lymphocytes
white Caucasians, testicular
  cancer 110

women
  and avoidable/unavoidable
    cancers 96
  breast cancer screening 136–7,
    137–8
  breast cancer statistics 104
  hormones and risk of breast
    cancer 103–9
  infection with HPV 93
  smoking and lung cancer
    mortality rates 67–8

X-rays
  and screening for colon
    cancer 142
  discovery 87
  sensitivity of AT carriers
    to 198
  In therapy 144
  see also mammography
    screening
xeroderma pigmentosa
  (XP) *118*, 121–2, 197

Yervoy™ 160
young people
  cervical cancer 93
  exposure to sunlight and skin
    cancer rates 82
  increase in smoking rates of 67
  teenagers infected with mono
    (glandular fever) 91, 192
  (*see also* children)